SO-ARE-928

Praise for *Oh, Baby!*

"I love this book. The chapter on Tia constantly taking pregnancy tests—that was me. I wanted it really badly. Congratulations, Tia. Our little girl is all grown up."

—*Wendy Williams*

"As fans of Tia and Tamera know, Tia's pregnancy was, uh, memorable. . . . She relives some of her greatest moments in her refreshingly candid new book. Here, as in the show, Tia is the queen of Too Much Information (isn't that what we love about her?). . . . Your favorite mom-to-be will thank you for this one."

—*Essence*

"A fresh take on being a new mom . . . light and breezy, yet informative."

—*Ebony*

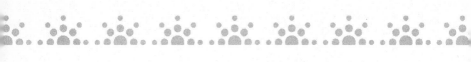

Tia Mowry

with Sheryl Berk

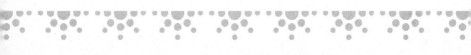

AVERY

a member of Penguin Group (USA) Inc.

New York

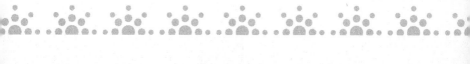

Oh, Baby!

Pregnancy Tales and Advice

from One Hot Mama

to Another

AVERY

Published by the Penguin Group
Penguin Group (USA) Inc., 375 Hudson Street,
New York, New York 10014, USA

USA · Canada · UK · Ireland · Australia
New Zealand · India · South Africa · China

Penguin Books Ltd, Registered Offices:
80 Strand, London WC2R 0RL, England
For more information about the Penguin Group visit penguin.com

First trade paperback edition 2013
Copyright © 2012 by Tia Mowry

All rights reserved. No part of this book may be reproduced, scanned, or distributed in any
printed or electronic form without permission. Please do not participate in or encourage piracy of
copyrighted materials in violation of the authors' rights. Purchase only authorized editions.
Published simultaneously in Canada

Unless otherwise noted, all photographs in insert courtesy Tia Mowry. Page 3, top left, courtesy
Tracy Blackwell. Page 4, all courtesy The Style Network © 2011 E! Entertainment LLC. Photographer:
Brandon Hickman. Page 5, top, courtesy Jose Villa; bottom right, courtesy Andrea Regalado.

Most Avery books are available at special quantity discounts for bulk purchase for sales promotions,
premiums, fund-raising, and educational needs. Special books or book excerpts also can be created to
fit specific needs. For details, write Penguin Group (USA) Inc. Special Markets, 375 Hudson Street,
New York, NY 10014.

The Library of Congress cataloged the hardcover edition as follows:

Mowry, Tia.
Oh, baby! : pregnancy tales and advice from one hot mama to another / Tia Mowry.
p.   cm.
ISBN 978-1-58333-482-9 (hardback)
1. Mowry Tia—Health.   2. Pregnancy—Popular works.   3. Pregnancy—Humor.
4. Childbirth—United States—Biography.   I. Title.
RG556.M69   2012   2011052353
618'.20092—dc23
[B]

ISBN 978-1-58333-528-4 (paperback edition)

Printed in the United States of America
1   3   5   7   9   10   8   6   4   2

BOOK DESIGN BY NICOLE LAROCHE

The "Ask the OB" sections are the result of Tia's own research and experience, and are based on the questions
she asked her own physician. They are not a substitute for seeking your own medical supervision. All matters
regarding your health require medical supervision. Neither the authors nor the publisher shall be liable or
responsible for any loss or damage allegedly arising from any information or suggestion in this book.

The recipes contained in this book are to be followed exactly as written. The publisher is not responsible for
your specific health or allergy needs that may require medical supervision. The publisher is not responsible
for any adverse reactions to the recipes contained in this book.

While the authors have made every effort to provide accurate telephone numbers, Internet addresses, and other
contact information at the time of publication, neither the publisher nor the authors assume any responsibility
for errors, or for changes that occur after publication. Further, the publisher does not have any control over and
does not assume any responsibility for author or third-party websites or their content.

Penguin is committed to publishing works of quality and integrity.
In that spirit, we are proud to offer this book to our readers;
however, the story, the experiences, and the words
are the author's alone.

CONTENTS

I want to dedicate this book

to my loving and supportive husband,

Cory Hardrict, and my joy and reason,

Cree Taylor Hardrict.

INTRODUCTION

I'm pregnant! What does that mean? Well, let's just state the obvious: I have a bun in the oven and I'm gonna be a mother. Someone's mama. A role model, a rule maker, a caregiver, the commander in chief. Bigger than Big Bird, you betcha, when it comes to a little person's life.

If you've picked up this book, you're probably in the same situation. Congrats! Whether you were pleasantly surprised or it's been a long journey (it certainly has been for me), welcome to the club. Go ahead; give yourself a pat on the back and a thunderous round of applause. Not everyone can do this (guys, for example). I don't know about you, but I feel like Superwoman. The power! The head rush! I feel like I could do anything: climb mountains, swim oceans, run with the bulls . . .

But I should warn you: This baby bliss won't last forever. For me, it started to wind down when I couldn't see my toes, keep food down, stop farting, or find anything to wear that would fit me besides a small tent. No, I was not feelin' like Ms. Fabulous in those moments. (And, lucky me, they were televised for the whole world to see on my reality show.) But that was when I told myself that when it sucks, I'll just laugh. I'll laugh even when I feel more like screaming or crying or strangling my husband for knocking me up. Because you have to keep things in perspective and keep your sense of humor when the world around you is spinning out of control.

Will I screw up? Absolutely. Will I break down? Several times a day. But in the end, I am the Queen of All Things (and my hormones are raging, so you better agree . . .). And so are you. You're the boss. Not your husband (sorry, honey), not your mother-in-law, not your well-meaning best girlfriend who wants you to give birth in a bathtub. *You* decide how this pregnancy is going to go, how you want to deliver your baby (barring any medical emergency), whether you want to breast-feed or go with formula (my boobs, my rules, I always say). Sometimes I feel like my head is going to explode, with all the information that is being shoved in my face. My advice? You take what feels right, what works for you, and leave the rest behind. Start listening to your developing mama instinct. Yes, you should be well informed and know your options, but in the end, you follow your gut. And trust me . . . by the time you hit the second trimester, that gut is hard to miss.

This book is not meant to stress you out or dictate what you should do. It's my take on my journey, from month one to delivery and beyond! It's the questions I asked my OB and the strategies I used to cope with every situation that arose, expected and unexpected, in the hope that what I have been through and learned along the way can help you. You too can hide your burgeoning belly from coworkers for several months, tell well-meaning moms to keep their opinions to themselves (politely!), and stifle the urge to puke every time you smell food, all while looking sexy as you grow to the size of a small semi-truck. I did it, and my experiences may not be yours (hopefully, you won't have as much gas), but every woman goes through her own adventure en route to mommyhood. Mentally, physically, and emotionally, it's a roller coaster—that explains the nausea. I hope to help you get through it with dignity and style.

And you're not alone. I am in it with you. I admit that despite my bravado, I was scared out of my mind from day one. I actually find it hysterically funny that people call it *expecting*, because I had no idea what to expect! How could I, when I know *nothing* about babies and pregnancy? I haven't done this before. Ever. And mind you, they don't teach Surviving Pregnancy 101 in college. If they did, we'd all probably be too scared to sign up for it. I am not one of those mothers who has been preparing to give birth since she was two. I was focusing on my education and my career. I'm learning as I go along. I'm winging it, big-time.

And soon enough, I'll be stronger, wiser, and watching *The Wiggles*. I'm okay with it. All of it. Because in the end, I'm going to have a brand-new baby boy and I will be able to say, *I did it. I rock. I am Mama—hear me roar!*

Are You Prepared to Be a Mom?

Well, you bought this book, so you'd better be! Or at least be up for the challenge! Answer True or False to the following statements, then check your score below.

1. Only wimps need sleep. *false*
2. I prefer watching *Barney* over *The Real Housewives*. *false*
3. I could change a diaper with one hand, hanging upside down, with my eyes closed. *true*
4. I know that *Yo Gabba Gabba!* is *not* Spanish for "I like to gossip..." *false*
5. Showers are totally overrated. *false*
6. I could stand to gain a few pounds... like, seventy. *false*
7. Eau de Spit-up would make a lovely perfume. *false*
8. I know what a Boppy is and I'm not afraid to use it. *false*
9. I'm totally psyched to taste strained peas. *false*
10. I'm cool with never again having (a) a minute to myself, (b) boobs that defy gravity, and (c) sex with my husband. *false*

If you answered True to all or most of the above, then, congrats—you are either a hundred percent ready to be a mother, or you cheated on this quiz.

If you answered False to all or most of the above, welcome to the thrilling, terrifying, totally bizarre world of pregnancy and motherhood. You're in the same boat that I was in—namely, you're clueless and trying to cram everything you need to know into the next nine months.

I thought I was a quick study—but this stuff is tough and sometimes deceiving.

Case in point: "You're registering for a Diaper Genie, right?" a friend asked me early in my pregnancy.

"You mean a big blue dude who will show up in my nursery and wipe my baby's butt for me? Sign me up!"

It's a lot to take in—I won't lie. But in the end, you'll be an expert in all things having to do with your baby. And one of the things you'll discover along the way is that a Diaper Genie is a garbage can that twists your kid's Pampers into a little sausage link that doesn't stink. Seriously—how cool is that?

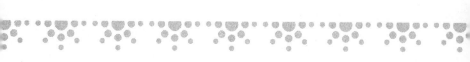

CHAPTER 1

Knocked Up . . . Kinda

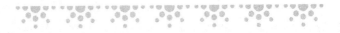

Every mama has a story of how she arrived at this moment. Some women are lucky: their hubbies just look at them and, bada bing—preggers. Not me. I never do anything the easy way. My path to pregnancy was no walk in the park . . .

*I*t all started when I was eighteen—not the trying-to-get-pregnant part (oh, my mama would have killed me!—not to mention that Disney and ABC might have, after they had kindly employed me as half of an adorable twin duo), but the endometriosis part. For those of you who don't know what endometriosis is—it's a royal pain in the gut and the butt. But if you want me to get all technical: according to the Endometriosis Association, endometriosis is a condition in which the tissue that lines and is shed by the uterus each month during menstruation grows in other areas of the body, causing pain, irregular bleeding, and, possibly, infertility. Translation: horrendous cramps. So bad that I had to excuse myself from my college classes to sit on the toilet for hours, whimpering and cursing. At the time, I figured that was what cramps during your period felt like. But it got worse.

Some years afterward, when I was in my late twenties, I was having my period, and I was doubled over with severe cramps. This time, it was so excruciating I thought I should call an ambulance. My husband, Cory, and I were engaged at the time, and I was really freaking him out. Men are not very good, if you don't already know, when it comes to anything gyno-related. They get that it happens once a month—and that it's messy, painful, and a relatively dangerous time to do anything that might piss us off, but that's about it. Most of them (including Cory) prefer to stay away. Far away.

But this time, I was really in agony. We both agreed I should probably at least call my doctor and ask what he thought I should do. Well, he had tons of advice on how to relieve the pain! He told me to get on the treadmill and walk (oh yeah, when you're in pain, *walking* is just what you want to do!), get in the tub, ice my stomach, and put heat on it. Nothing worked. I was wet, cold, hot, and pacing at the same time. One of my friends in our building helped me get an appointment with a gynecologist, Dr. Dolores Kent. She delivered Jada Pinkett Smith's kids, so I knew she had the creds. I also liked the idea that I could bump into Will Smith in the waiting room one day.

Dr. Kent examined me, listened to my tale of woe, and told me she thought I had endometriosis. *Thought*—as in: "No, I'm not positive. I'm a doctor, not a psychic." It turns out the only way you can be a hundred percent sure you have endometriosis is to have surgery and check it out. Dr. Kent explained the procedure: She would make a small incision in my stomach and actually go through my belly button with a camera probe. Then she'd take a peek around in there and see what was causing the pain. It all sounded very *Alien* to me. And while I have spent most of my life in front of a camera, I was not too eager to have my internal organs on a big screen. I should also add that I am a total scaredy-cat. Scalpels, needles, anesthesia, paper cuts . . . they freak me out. Plus, there was also the very real possibility that it *wasn't* endometriosis—maybe I just had a low pain threshold and some raging PMS every month. Then this surgery would be just for the fun of it.

"Look, Tia," Dr. Kent said. "If it *is* endometriosis, it's going to be hard to have a baby." I let those words sink in for a few moments. I was getting married and we wanted to eventually start a family. Exactly *how* hard would it be?

"Hard," she replied. The way she said it and the grave look on her face made me hear it more like "Virtually impossible." So I agreed to the surgery—scared to death as I was to be (a) knocked out and (b) cut open. Luckily, as Dr. Kent promised, it wasn't painful or a huge ordeal. It did turn out to be endometriosis. Besides poking that little camera around my uterus and ovaries, the doctors were able to scrape away the scar tissue, so the pain during my periods lessened almost immediately. I hoped that when we were ready to become parents, we'd have no problem. Case closed.

But two and a half years later, the pain started getting bad again. I realized just how bad it was while I was in a meeting with my manager and my sister, Tamera, pitching an animated series. We were talking about making ourselves into cartoons, and suddenly I was writhing in pain. Tamera looked at me: "Again?"

Yup, again. I went back to the doctor, and she confirmed that the endometriosis was back. Lucky me. Along with the physical pain came the confusion and fear of not knowing whether my body would be able to carry a child. Cory and I were ready to have a baby. At this point, we had been married for a year and a half, and together for about eleven years—it felt like it was time. It had taken a while for me to get to this point, too. I always knew I wanted a child, but for so long, my career was my number-one priority. I had been a child star and I wanted to make a comeback, and after finishing college, I dove right back into acting. I took classes, hired a trainer—the whole nine yards. The last thing on my mind was getting pregnant.

Cory, however, constantly talked babies from the day we got married, April 20, 2008. He really wanted to be a dad bad! He's a natural nurturer; it's one of the qualities that made me fall in love with him. His entire family lives in Chicago, and it was just us two in L.A. He wanted to start a family of our own here. But I stood my ground. Not yet. I wasn't ready.

"I guess I'm going to have to take matters into my own hands and adopt a child, since you're not going to give me one," he would tease. Even though he said it jokingly, I knew he was serious. I could see it in his eyes.

"Just think about it?" He made me promise.

As *The Game*'s ratings grew and my career began moving along again, I finally told Cory I'd give it some serious thought. But how does one go about making one of the biggest decisions of her life? I watched young moms pushing strollers down the street. They were so happy, so nurturing. I could do that, I told myself. I closed my eyes and pictured myself rocking an infant in my arms and singing a lullaby. And just like that, I had it: baby fever. The sight of a mom kissing her child made me go all mushy. I wanted one of those, too! Cory was overjoyed when I told him I was ready. That was when we were hit with the *E* word, *endometriosis*, and my best-laid plans fell apart. We had been trying for a year, and nada. Considering the pain I was in and my dreams of becoming a mother, Dr. Kent advised me to have a second surgery.

After the surgery, Cory and I started trying again, and I began to research what was happening in my body. I wanted to know why the endometriosis kept recurring. My doctor recommended—if I didn't want to wind up in the hospital again—that I change my diet. At the suggestion of my friend and *Game* costar Brittany Daniel, I started the Body Ecology Diet. The diet teaches you how to eat to reduce inflammation in the body that (among other things) can contribute to endometriosis. But when I first heard about it, I thought it was a bunch of mumbo jumbo. Couldn't I go on a cookie diet or something, and see if that worked? It sounded so much simpler, and tastier!

Brittany wouldn't take no for an answer: "Tia, just go get the book." I did. I read it and tried it, for an entire year. In the beginning it was torture. You eat 80 percent vegetables, 20 percent protein, no juices, no processed sugar, and no carbs. I grew up in a southern family. The staples of my pre–Body Ecology Diet had been real southern classics—like Paula Deen's versions of smothered mashed potatoes, mac and cheese, and fried chicken (I own all her cookbooks!). I also love Italian food: spaghetti and meatballs, garlic bread dripping in butter. My mom would cook these favorites for me, and I would cook them for Cory. When I started the diet, my body was screaming, "Hey, what is going on here? Where are the grits? Where's the linguini?" But after a while it got easier and I started to feel more energetic. I also got really skinny (another plus!). I was doing yoga every day and eating healthy—I was in my best shape ever and feeling great.

And then something even better happened. I was in Atlanta, shooting *The Game* and staying in a hotel. I felt weird. I didn't know how to describe it, other than that I was spacey and exhausted. Cory was away shooting a movie in Canada, and I called him.

"Honey, I think I'm pregnant."

"Tia." My poor husband sighed. "You *always* think you're pregnant." He was right. I did tend to jump the gun. At least half a dozen times before, I had been *positive* I was preggers, only to discover it was indigestion.

"No, this time I mean it," I insisted. "Hang on, honey, I'm going to test right now." I pulled out a digital pregnancy tester—which I had been carrying around for a while now, just in case. Lo and behold . . . it was positive. I started jumping up and down in my hotel room, crying.

I thought Cory was in shock. "Honey? Did you hear what I said?" I snapped a picture on my phone of the pregnancy stick and sent it to him. But he wasn't astonished: he just didn't believe it. I was like the boy who cried wolf, only in my case I was the girl who cried pregnant. I started to doubt it myself—maybe the digital thingamajig was wrong. Maybe I should go get a few old-school kits and try them.

The next day I went to the store and picked up a traditional EPT. The little blue line popped up in the window: *pregnant*. But we weren't celebrating yet. I think we were just so nervous, after trying for a year and seeing nothing happen, that now, even

though we had the news we'd been waiting for, it was still hard
to believe. "I think I need a real medical opinion," I told Cory.
I went to the emergency room. There, an intern tested me and
cheerfully told me, "Nope. You're not pregnant." I wanted to
strangle the guy.

"What? Dude, no, I took a test. I took two of them. They
both said I was pregnant. You are outnumbered!"

But the doc was not wavering. "*This* test says you're not
pregnant."

I could not get him to budge—he was not going to let me
have this.

I went back to my hotel, devastated, but there was a thought
still nagging at me: Doctors can screw up. I've watched my fair
share of *Grey's Anatomy*. Not even McDreamy is a hundred percent on his game all the time. Maybe this McDowner was wrong,
too. Maybe I *was* pregnant and he just didn't know it.

Six more EPTs later, the evidence was mounting—literally.
I pleaded with my husband. "Cory, I am telling you, all these
sticks can't be wrong." I even snapped a picture of one of the
boxes—"99 percent accurate!"—and sent it to him.

Finally, I got an appointment with an OB in Atlanta who
performed a sonogram. I held my breath. There, on the monitor, was a tiny dark circle—the yolk sac. Validation! I was pregnant! But before I could leap off the exam table and do the
happy dance, the OB warned me that sometimes when you have
endometriosis, you can have an ectopic pregnancy, which occurs
outside the womb and has to be terminated. She told me I had
to wait a few more weeks to see if there was a heartbeat.

I felt like I was on this crazy emotional roller coaster—yes,

I'm pregnant; no, I'm not; maybe I am. I thought you could never be "a little pregnant."

"Let's just be cautiously optimistic," I told Cory. I was scared to death. I was afraid if I held on to any hope, I'd jinx it.

Three weeks later, I returned to the OB for another sonogram. Cory was still away and I hadn't told anyone what was going on. In fact, I told my production team I had a doctor's appointment for gastro issues. It was the first of my many fertility fibs. (If you think you'll need help with those, see "Excuses, Excuses!" in chapter 2.) I was shaking in the stirrups, as the doctor slathered my stomach in cold blue gel and then rolled the Doppler around trying to get a picture. There was silence . . . then a flicker on the screen. A heartbeat! The doc congratulated me. I was officially pregnant. I could barely wrap my brain around it.

Ask the OB

My doctor Layne Kumetz, M.D., FACOG (Fellow of the American College of Obstetricians and Gynecologists), is *amazing*. She's young, vibrant, and full of personality. She kept me calm from day one to the Big Day (not an easy task, I assure you) and encouraged me to ask any question that popped into my head—no matter how stupid, bizarre, or embarrassing. After she listened to me moan and groan for nine months (including middle-of-the-night panicked phone calls!), I trusted her implicitly. I knew she would look out for me and my baby, take every precaution, and steer me in the right direction. In these boxes, I will share the very real questions I asked her, and her answers, which I hope will be helpful to you.

Okay, the initial shock (I'm preggers!) is over. What should I do?

Whether or not you've taken a home pregnancy test, go see your doctor. A urine sample will be taken to formally confirm you are pregnant. Assuming you are feeling relatively well, you should schedule your first visit with your ob-gyn about 6 to 7 weeks after the first day of your last period. Your due date will be established based on your last period and/or by an ultrasound. If you are having unusual symptoms, such as spotting or severe abdominal pain, you should be evaluated sooner. Discuss with your doctor any medical conditions as well as all over-the-counter or prescription medications you are taking.

Some other things to put into effect as soon as you find out, all having to do with preventing birth defects: Stop smoking, taking drugs, and drinking alcohol right away; ask for help if you need it. Be sure you are getting 400 to 800 micrograms of folic acid every day. Avoid contact with toxic substances or materials at work or at home that could be harmful. Stay away from cat litter boxes—it's time for Daddy-to-be to assume that chore.

> How much weight will I gain with my pregnancy,
> and how long will it take to get it off?
>
> If you are starting out at a healthy weight, I would expect you to
> gain about twenty-five pounds over the next nine months. It's
> important not to gain too much weight, because that's not
> healthy for you or the baby, and it will take longer to lose. You
> need to eat only about 300 extra calories per day, compared
> with your pre-pregnancy diet. So, contrary to popular advice
> from well-meaning grandmothers, you are not "eating for two"
> when you are pregnant. How long it will take to lose the weight
> depends a little on how much you gain and whether or not you
> plan to breast-feed. Post-delivery you can expect to lose about
> five pounds per month with regular exercise.

Start Spreading the News

I always fantasized about how I would break the news to my
husband. You know, those corny things people do: baby rattles,
a "Dad" T-shirt, balloons, and so on. I couldn't do any of this
for Cory. I couldn't even give him a hug, because we were working about nine hundred miles away from each other. But he
didn't mind: he was over the moon when I called him from the
doctor's office. And once we got the thumbs-up from the doc
at twelve weeks, we decided it would be okay to let a few friends

and family members in on it. But one other person got the news as soon as we knew. The first person I called after my hubby was my best friend, Jessica Laskey. I've known her since I was twelve, and I tell her everything. We sounded like teenagers on the phone.

"Can you believe it?" I squealed.

"No! I can't believe it! This is amazing! How did it happen?"

I giggled. "Do you want me to tell you about the birds and the bees?"

What she meant was how we had managed to get pregnant after everything I had gone through with my endometriosis.

"It must be God's timing. I am so happy," I told her. And she was elated for me, though in shock for several days. If I had told her in person, I would have pinched her.

I kept my mom in the dark till about eight weeks. I knew telling her would be a huge deal. In case the pregnancy was ectopic, I didn't want to disappoint her. You have to understand, Mama had been on our case from day one for Cory and me to give her a grandchild: "Wait much longer and your father and I are going to be ancient or dead," she reminded me. I knew I had to be sure before I told her all that nagging had finally paid off.

I called and braced myself for her reaction. "You're going to be extremely excited . . ." I began.

No sooner had I gotten out the words "I'm pregnant" than she started bawling. My mom may seem like a tough lady—she was an army drill sergeant, after all—but she has the biggest heart. And when it comes to babies, that big ol' heart melts. So she cried and cried and cried . . . for days. Less than a month before, she'd lost her brother to cancer, and the news of a new life coming into the family in the middle of all this loss made her so happy.

There was just one catch. "You can't tell Dad, or Tamera, or Tavior, or Tahj," I warned her. I didn't want my father or siblings to hear it from anyone but me, and I wanted to wait till the twelve-week mark, when I had more assurance the baby would be okay.

Not being able to blab for a whole month drove her absolutely nuts. Sorry, Mama! I know I gave her gray hairs with this assignment. But I especially wanted to tell Tamera in person. We're so close, and I wanted to see her face, feel her excitement. We hadn't seen each other for two weeks, and I couldn't wait for her to visit me in Atlanta.

As soon as she arrived, I sat her down in my hotel room. "Sissy, I have some good news and some bad news."

She leaned forward. "What's up?"

"The good news is I'm pregnant. The bad news is I'm going to be very pregnant at your wedding." Poor Tamera: her matron of honor would be the size of a blimp, probably blocking most of the wedding party in her pics. I also wasn't sure bridesmaid dresses came in tent sizes.

"It's fine! I knew it!" she cried, hugging me.

"You knew? How did you know? Did Mom blab?"

"Come on, Tia! I'm your twin. We were in the womb together. I knew from the moment you said, 'Sit down.'" We cried and hugged some more, and marveled at our twin telepathy. I was so glad I told her in person. I will always remember the look on my sis's face: the laughter, the tears of joy, the "You can't pull one over on me" smirk. "I'm going to be an auntie!" she said, beaming.

Once I started telling people, it was hard to hold myself back. You'll probably feel the same way, like you want to take out a billboard: "Look, y'all, I'm having a baby!" Funnily enough, the Style Network actually did it for me. Shortly before I delivered, they put a ginormous *Tia & Tamera* billboard in Times Square. There I was, nine months pregnant, like some jolly, fat giant looming over New York City! In case anyone in the metropolitan area missed the articles in *People* or *Us Weekly*, you knew now: Tia Mowry is preggers . . . big-time!

Before *you* blurt out the news, I strongly recommend that you consider the timing that is right for you. For me, I needed some reassurance that I was out of "the danger zone." Everything was going well, and the baby was okay. I have lots of friends who are superstitious and didn't want to say anything till they absolutely had to (like, when they could no longer wear anything but maternity clothes). As a guideline, I think it's fine to share the news with one very close friend or family member the first month. By the end of the first trimester, it's fine to tell family and close friends. By the middle of the second trimester, you can share the news with bosses, close colleagues, and work friends, and let the news spread by word of blabbermouths. After that, I say go ahead and blog about it, post on Facebook, however you want to get the word out in a big way. Or don't—you can always wait till you have a beautiful new baby pic to share the news with the world.

So . . . What Are You Having?
How to Tell Your Baby's Gender

I told myself I didn't care what sex our baby was—all I wanted was a healthy infant. But to be completely honest, I was curious. I hated the idea of referring to our baby as It until the 18-to-20-week ultrasound. Couldn't I just have a hint? There are all kinds of theories on how you can tell. Consider the following as you count down the weeks until you know. None is 100 percent accurate, but they are definitely fun ways to pass the time.

Perfect timing: This theory says you'll have a boy if you had sex 24 hours before ovulation and a girl if you got horizontal 2 to 4 days before ovulation. This theory is based on the fact that female sperm (the X chromosome) live longer than male sperm and swim slower. So if you had sex a few days before you ovulated, it's more likely that it was a female sperm that was still hanging around.

You're carrying high (or low): This old wives' tale states that if you're carrying high, buy pink. If your bump is low, you're carrying a boy. Total strangers would come up to me on the street and declare, "You're having a boy," judging from the way I carried. For a long time, I looked like I had swallowed a basketball—my bump just hovered somewhere around my belly button. I've had friends who carried low and had girls, but it was telling for me.

Oh, Baby!

Beat still, my heart: When your OB uses the Doppler to listen to the baby's heartbeat, ask for the heart rate. Some people believe that 140-plus beats per minute indicates a girl, and below 140 a boy.

Girls are sweet: At least according to this rumor. Supposedly, if you crave sweet treats while pregnant, you'll have a baby girl. If you prefer salty or sour: a boy's on board. Yeah, this one was true for me.

Ancient Chinese secret: The Chinese gender-predictor chart uses your age and conception month to predict if you are having a boy or a girl. The results are supposedly more than 90 percent accurate. (I tried it, and it was correct!) See babygenderprediction.com/chinese-gender-chart.html.

The ring trick: Tie a plain, round ring (like a wedding band) to a string. Hang it over your belly. If it swings in a circle, a boy's in your future. If it goes back and forth, you've got a girl.

Face facts: Your face looks round (moonfaced), tired, or blemished—congrats, it's a girl! Supposedly, a girl steals her mom's beauty. I dunno, I looked like crap most of the time, and I gave birth to a boy.

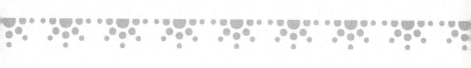

CHAPTER 2

Who, Me? Preggers?

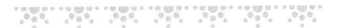

I went from wanting to shout, "I'm havin' a baby!" from the rooftops, to thinking, Oh, crap, no one can know! My character on The Game, Melanie Barnett, is a vixen, not a soccer mom. Funny how I never really thought about it till now—this could be a big problem at work . . .

I was working twelve to fifteen hours every day and throwing up constantly. By week three I had to keep excusing myself to the bathroom to hurl. It's a joke that they call it morning sickness; I had it in the afternoon, at night, and every minute in between.

One of our producers, Mara Brock Akil, was concerned. She took me aside and whispered, "Tia, is there a problem?"

Uh-oh . . . had she heard me barfing in the bathroom?

"Problem?" I played totally dumb, praying another wave of nausea didn't hit me while we were chatting. She had on really nice shoes . . .

"You know, over the past year you've lost some weight, and now you're going to the bathroom a lot . . ." Mara began.

Oh, that kind of problem. Mara didn't think I was pregnant. She thought I was sticking my finger down my throat. What a relief!

"No, really, it's not that. I just have some gastro issues," I lied. "I'm okay."

Mara raised an eyebrow. "Really?"

I smiled. "Absolutely! Now, if you could excuse me . . . I need to run to the ladies' room."

I managed to keep my little secret until about the eighth week of my pregnancy. At that point, the jig was up. *The Game* is a very sexy show, and I am in lingerie half the time on camera. I didn't think I was showing, but people began to whisper that I looked like I might be packing on some extra pounds around my middle. (Yes, I could hear you . . .) The wardrobe stylist couldn't understand how my bra size had suddenly shot up a full cup, or why the outfits I had worn six weeks before were suddenly impossible to zip.

"Oh, it's just gas," I said, smiling.

I used my "gastrointestinal issue" to explain my fifty trips to the bathroom every day. I had been hospitalized twice for dehydration (morning sickness can do that to you), so it was plausible that I had a nasty case of diarrhea. People on set would look at me weird: I was a getting a rep as the Chick with the Poop Problem. Most of them bought it or just didn't want to hear all the gory details. Humiliating? Yes. But what would be worse, I told myself, was if they knew I was pregnant. I worried I'd be out of a job. When you've been acting since you were a kid, you learn the harsh reality: Show business is just a business. And a pregnant actress doing a love scene in a bra and panties is not exactly an asset. Especially if her ass-et is growing daily!

But emotionally, keeping the news to myself was killing me. I wanted to get it off my chest, so two months into my pregnancy I decided it was time to tell. My cast mates were first. I wanted to tell them individually to get their reactions—might as well have some fun with this!

The first person I told was Coby Bell, who plays wide receiver Jason Pitts. I knew he would understand. He has a family of four already—two sets of twins! He's very sensitive and family-oriented; I knew I'd get the support from him. Besides, he was always telling me, "Tia, do it! Do it! Have a kid!"

"I'm pregnant," I told him quietly.

"Yes!" he cheered, pumping his fist in the air. That was just the enthusiasm I needed to propel me forward. Brittany Daniel, who plays Coby's wife and my friend on the show, was the second person I filled in and she was also thrilled: "I knew the diet would help!" she said, hugging me. She also resisted the urge (thank you, Brit!) to say, "Told ya so!"

Then I told Wendy Raquel Robinson, a.k.a. Tasha Mack, mother and manager of the Sabers' star quarterback, Malik Wright, on *The Game*. A coworker and close friend, she's been married awhile and we have confided in each other as married women. Now I was excited to share my big news with her!

"Oh my God, I'm so happy for you," she said—but I could see she was kind of in a state of disbelief. And from that day on, she was afraid to touch my belly!

Hosea Chanchez, who plays Malik, was my next victim. He's the party guy on the set; I didn't know how he'd react.

"You can't come out clubbing with us anymore—and you're more fun when you're drunk!" he teased. Well, he did have a point. But I promised him, preggers or not, I knew how to par-tay!

The last cast member I told was Pooch Hall, otherwise known

to *Game* fans as Derwin Davis. Well, technically, Pooch guessed. I was waiting to tell him at the end of production, because I didn't want it to affect our chemistry on the show—he plays my love interest. We were in front of the entire crew, rehearsing a scene, when he blurted it out.

"Oh my God, Tia! Are you pregnant?" he gasped, patting my tummy. Pooch actually noticed I had a pooch! I shushed him and pulled him aside.

"Yeah, I'm pregnant. Could you not tell the world?" I pleaded.

He hugged me and grinned. "I'm gonna call you Mama T from now on."

So all in all, it took about a week to break the news to my costars. There were tears; there were screams; there were hugs; even a few "Are you kidding me?" responses. Then I decided it was time to let executive producer Salim Akil in on the big news. I figured he had a hunch—he had spotted me sleeping on set in between takes and making frequent trips to the bathroom. I was planning how I would say it when he suddenly called me into a room for a sit-down. I started sweating bullets.

"Tia, what is going on?" he asked.

"I, um, well, you see . . . I'm having a baby." (I neglected to add, "Oh, and sorry if this is a huge pain in the butt for our show—I know my timing stinks.")

I braced myself for his reaction. Would he freak? Yell? Pass out?

Instead, he leaned in and gave me a huge hug. "I am thrilled for you!" he said. I was thrilled, too. Thrilled that the cat was finally out of the bag. Thrilled everyone knew that I had a bun in the oven and wasn't binge eating. I couldn't have asked for a more supportive group of friends and colleagues.

Excuses, Excuses!

How to Keep Your Pregnancy Under Wraps Until You're Ready to Reveal It

This is so much easier if the smell of food doesn't make you gag and you're not peeing every three minutes. Some ladies are lucky not to show at all. Case in point: Until she delivered, did anyone suspect Nicole Kidman was actually preggers? It's also harder to hide (I hear) after baby number one. You pop a lot sooner. But here are some tried-and-true tips on how to keep your business to yourself when inquiring minds wanna know.

Scenario 1: Your gossipy coworker corners you at the water cooler and asks, "Have you put a little weight on—or are you pregnant?"

How to handle it: Better she thinks you're fat—so look embarrassed and reply, "Yes, I have, in fact, put on a few pounds. I've found this amazing new fro-yo place with sixteen flavors on my block, and I am determined to try every one of them." Or better yet—say nothing. Stuff a Snickers bar in your face and shrug!

Scenario 2: Your sister-in-law spies "OB" in red on your calendar and demands to know your due date.

How to handle it: Laugh and brush it off. "No, no . . . OB stands for Outward Bound! Didn't I tell you? I volunteered to take our local high school teens on a white-water rafting trip." Another option: "Heavens, no! I just have a nasty itch down there and I need to get it checked out." That should shut her up.

Scenario 3: Your boss calls you into her office. She's heard rumors that you're expecting.

How to handle it: Keep calm and cool and reply, "Expecting? Yes, I'm expecting a Federal Express delivery today. Gotta go track it online!" Another good retort: "You know, I think the gossip in this office is very counterproductive. I volunteer to find out who is spreading these rumors and give you a full report first thing in the morning!"

Scenario 4: You go out to lunch with your girlfriend and the smell of her baked cod makes you turn green.

How to handle it: Excuse yourself to the little girls' room (hopefully till she finishes her entire entrée), then explain, "The news said there's a vicious stomach bug going around," or "Sorry, I had to take an important business call from my boss."

Scenario 5: Your BFF catches you reading an issue of *Fit Pregnancy* on the beach and wants to know "Whassup with that?"

How to handle it: Resist the urge to bury the mag in the sand—looks way too guilty. Instead, tell her there's a fascinating article about hemorrhoids on page 30—would she like to see some photos? If she's still not buying, point out some hunk's greased-up biceps on the beach and change the subject *fast*.

Spilling the Beans

When you are ready for the big reveal, there are better ways than others to do it.

DON'T . . .

- Tell acquaintances or strangers *before* family. Your mother-in-law will never speak to you again if she hears it from the mailman.
- Show up for work in a T-shirt that reads "Knocked Up."
- Spell it out in gummy letters or Alpha-Bits.
- Send out a mass e-mail with photos of your blooming belly. Have we learned nothing from Anthony Weiner?
- Assume people will figure it out without your telling them. I swear, I was a week away from my delivery date

and I had a woman look at my huge stomach and ask me, "Are you pregnant?" I wanted to reply, "Nah, I'm trying to get on that *Biggest Loser* show . . ."

DO . . .

- Be creative. Take your mom out to lunch and present to her a little baby onesie that says "I love Grandma!" or give your sis a box of tampons with the note "I won't be needing these for nine months." You can also snap a pic of your positive EPT test and make it your Facebook photo.

- Expect the unexpected: a macho-guy friend who bursts into tears; a coworker who is not as excited (now she'll have to absorb your workload while you're on maternity leave!); a college roommate who gives you the cold shoulder. Basically, it's their issue, not yours. You're happy. Don't let anyone burst your bubble with a bad vibe. But *do* be sensitive to a pal who might be dealing with infertility. I know firsthand the stress/heartbreak of trying to get pregnant while everyone around you is expecting. It sucks. As happy as I was for these friends, it did hurt a bit to hear of someone's pregnancy when we were trying unsuccessfully for a year. Be kind.

- If it's a holiday (Christmas, Valentine's Day, Easter) or a birthday, send cards for grandparents, aunts, and uncles. Your family will get the message!

- Say it with a song: Take your friends and family out for a night of karaoke. Perform a duet with your hubby to a tune with "Baby" in the title to hint at the news: Mariah Carey's "Always Be My Baby," Justin Bieber's "Baby," even Sir Mix-A-Lot's "Baby Got Back"!

Tell Me More, Tell Me More

What should you share and what should you keep to yourself? I had to learn this the hard way. During an interview with *Parents* magazine, the reporter asked me what the hardest part about being pregnant was. "Oh, that's easy," I volunteered. "I used to throw up and poop at the same time! It just all came out at once, you know?" There was a long silence, then, "No, I didn't know. I didn't *need* to know. It's okay—you don't have to go into such detail . . ." I was mortified. I had grossed the interviewer out! Before you say what's on your mind, answer Y or N to the following, then check your answers below.

	Y/N
1. The sex of the baby	Y
2. Your registry gift list	Y
3. Your birth plan	N
4. Your bra size	N
5. How many pints of Ben & Jerry's you scarfed down last night	N
6. The fact that you rub extra-virgin olive oil on your thighs every night to prevent stretch marks	N
7. Your OB's contact info	Y

8. How and where you conceived   N
9. The naked pregnancy portrait à la Demi Moore you had taken   N
10. Your panic that delivering will hurt like hell   Y
11. What you're planning to name the baby   Y
12. Whether you're planning to breast-feed   Y
13. The crazy-ass erotic dream you had last night about you and Boris Kodjoe and a tub of Cool Whip   N
14. Every food that makes you want to puke   Y
15. The new sex position you had to try last night with your hubby since your belly was too big   N

Answers

1. **THE SEX OF THE BABY.** I was comfortable telling people I was carrying a boy. People tend to buy gender-neutral yellow onesies if they're not sure what you're having. I wanted blue! But like the fact that you're pregnant, it's really no one's beeswax until you want to tell.

2. **YOUR REGISTRY.** After "What are you having?" the next question people tend to ask is where you are registered. This is so they can buy, buy baby everything—so you don't have to. People are happy to have a hand in getting you ready for your big arrival, and this helpful hint can go out by word of mouth, e-mail, and printed on your shower invites. If you feel this is being too pushy, then have your sister do it (oh, Tamera . . .).

3. **YOUR BIRTH PLAN.** Tell the people who *should* know! You want your husband, your health care professional, and

your midwife or doula to understand *exactly* how you want this to go—and what your wishes are just in case it doesn't. It's not so much a plan as it is a list of preferences to help you envision what the Big Day will be like. I know this sounds silly, but let's just say you are otherwise occupied—i.e., screaming your head off in labor pains—and a nice nurse comes in and asks, "Would you like an epidural?" If you can't answer her, and have indicated that you want pain relief in your birth plan, then your hubby (hopefully!) will raise his hand high and yell, "Oh, yeah! Give it to her now!" so you can nod in agreement between moans. The plan should include who you want in the labor room (your hubby) and who you don't (your crazy aunt Ethel). It can also say what positions you'd like to be in for your labor—lying down, standing up, squatting—and if you want "assistance" in the birth, that is, forceps. Of course, realize none of this is written in stone. I was certain I was going to give birth naturally until my doctor informed me the baby was breech and I needed a C-section. Some things are going to be out of your control, and by then you'll have had nine months to get used to it. Your birth plan at least gives you an idea of how things might go.

Ask the OB

Doula, midwife, or delivery in hospital?
I'm so confused! How do I decide?

Assuming you are healthy and at low risk for complications, if you're looking for a practitioner who takes a more holistic approach to your care, a midwife may be a good option. That said, there are some physicians who provide this kind of personalized care, too, and some midwives who may not, so consider meeting a few different practitioners before making your decision.

Midwives traditionally have more time to answer all your questions and help you learn about the physical and emotional changes you experience throughout pregnancy. If you are going to go that route, it's important to seek out a certified nurse-midwife (CNM.) To be certified, a CNM must be formally educated through an accredited program and pass a rigorous national certifying exam. A doula is more like a labor coach, and can support women who are under the care of either a midwife or physician, but typically a doula is not able to perform the actual delivery.

One of the main differences between a midwife and a medical doctor is their training. In order to become an obstetrician, eight years of training are required after college. Physicians are trained to recognize and manage most complications and emergencies that may arise in the course of a pregnancy and delivery, and they can perform a cesarean section if necessary. A midwife is trained to manage normal, uncomplicated, low-risk pregnancies. If there are any complications with your pregnancy or delivery, your care will be transferred to an obstetrician. Here in the United States, between the two options, obstetricians are by far the most common choice, accounting for more than ninety percent of deliveries in 2006.

With regard to a home birth versus a hospital delivery, I cannot stress enough how strongly I encourage every woman to deliver in a hospital setting. Even a seemingly uncomplicated birth can still potentially become a life-threatening emergency without warning. I've seen postpartum hemorrhages in low-risk healthy women who likely wouldn't have made it to the hospital in time. I've also seen a newborn with an unexpected lung problem whose life was saved only by immediate resuscitative efforts and neonatal care. Although the absolute risk of planned home births is low, it does carry an increased, two- to threefold risk of newborn death when compared with planned hospital births. I would personally never consider giving birth at home. With a supportive delivery team, you can easily have a completely beautiful, loving, unmedicated delivery in the safe setting of a hospital, just in case your uterus or the baby decides not to follow the birth plan.

4. **YOUR BRA SIZE.** If the salesgirl at Victoria's Secret asks, by all means, share away. Maybe she'll find something you can fit into these days besides one of those over-the-shoulder boulder holders at maternity stores. I also rec-

ommend sharing your new boob measurement with your
hubby as foreplay. Mention the words "E-cup" and watch
his eyes light up . . . When it comes to cups, most pregnant women's runneth over. Pamela Anderson, eat your
heart out.

Ask the OB

How big are my boobs going to get when I'm pregnant?

Every woman is different, but one of the first signs of pregnancy
for many women is an increase in breast size. The increase in
hormone levels frequently leads to breast swelling and enlarge-
ment in the first trimester, and typically doesn't end there.
Cup size can continue to grow throughout the pregnancy.
Additionally, bra size may increase as well. During pregnancy
your lung capacity increases, expanding your rib cage and potentially resulting in a wider chest diameter. Investing in good
maternity bras early on can help minimize the expense of buying
new bras and then finding out they don't fit anymore as time
goes by.

5. **HOW MANY PINTS OF BEN & JERRY'S YOU SCARFED DOWN.**
Mum's the word on this one—no one but you and your
doctor need to know how crazy your cravings are getting.
Just keep the fridge stocked with plenty of replacements,
so your hubby isn't running to the store at two a.m.

6. **OLIVE OIL ON YOUR THIGHS.** Margarine on your hips. Cocoa butter on your boobs. Hey, whatever works—you wouldn't believe some of the stuff I tried. It's no one's business what you're doing to keep your bod beautiful as it becomes stretched and pulled like Silly Putty. If your friend asks you for your secret to glowing skin, tell her it's the hormones or Crème de la Mer, not Land O'Lakes.

7. **YOUR OB'S INFO.** Most women get very possessive of their OBs—I can't explain why, except to say we feel connected to these people and totally trust them. I knew I had bonded with Dr. Kumetz when she asked me one day, "How are *you* doing?" Every visit, all we had talked about was how the baby was—but she really wanted to know how I was feeling, physically and emotionally. She let me vent! She felt like a close friend and confidante—I hated to share her! However, it's important that your husband, close family member, or friend has the doctor's number in case of an emergency—for instance, if your water breaks while you're driving on the freeway.

8. **HOW AND WHERE YOU CONCEIVED.** That is a tough call. If it's some romantic story, such as you made a baby while making love on a starlit beach in St. Barts, I say, sure, spill—to your close friends. But if it was in the backseat of your dad's pickup truck or at thirty thousand feet in an airplane potty . . . pass. No one needs the dirty deets.

9. **YOUR "DEMI" PORTRAIT.** Unless you're an exhibitionist, you're probably not going to hang this one on your living room wall. More likely, these photos are for you and your husband to share and to remember this moment. If,

however, you think pregnancy is a beautiful thing and you love your body and all its curves, I see no prob in showing a few close friends and family the shots. Just ask before you show. You don't want to give your mother-in-law a heart attack, flashing your privates without preparing her first! My photographer, Dimitry, convinced me to pose in the buff during a magazine photo shoot. My publicist, Jordyn, said, "If you pose nude, they'll put you on the cover—like Britney Spears, Christina Aguilera, and Demi Moore." Hmmmm . . . I do love those covers! Cory was like, "I say do it! Go out with a bang! Can I get naked on the cover, too?" In the end, I wasn't comfortable publishing the pics right away. Instead, I framed one and gave it to Cory as a present.

10. **YOUR PANIC.** No one wants to admit they're terrified. But trust me when I tell you every pregnant woman has at least one "What have I gotten myself into?" moment. Mine happened the minute my doc mentioned the word "C-section." Total hysteria set in. And you know what? I felt a lot better once I talked to people about it. Most of my friends assured me it would be okay. They'd either been through it or knew someone who had. You don't have to be ashamed if you're scared to death to deliver. God knows I was . . . There! I said it!

11. **THE BABY'S NAME.** Sure, if you like, you can tell. But be prepared for people to try and convince you to change it, to look at you like you're nuts, or to make a disapproving face. I cannot tell you how many people scratched their heads when I told them we were naming our son Cree

Oh, Baby!

Taylor (for the record, the first name has Cory's initial, and the middle name has mine). It's your choice as a couple what you want you want to call your kid—be it Apple (à la Gwyneth Paltrow), Blanket (à la Michael Jackson), or Kumkwat. Okay, I just made that one up.

What's in a Name?

Regardless of all of the opinions, naming trends, and traditions that go into the decision you ultimately make, the overwhelming truth is that the name you call your kid will be the one he's stuck with all his life—and the one he has to live up to. It's a pretty serious decision and one you shouldn't make in haste. When Cory and I sat down to talk baby names, we knew we wanted to keep my family tradition of the baby's first name beginning with the first letter of the dad's name and the middle name beginning with the first letter of the mom's.

"Okay," I told my hubby, "we have C and T to work with."

Cory had a request as well: "I want the name to mean *warrior*." He's always wanted to get that word as a tattoo because he feels like he's been a warrior and a survivor all his life, and he's proud of it. His mom died at a young age from cancer, and when he came out here to L.A., he had only $100 in his pocket. "I fought so much to get where I am today," he told me. He wanted his son to be a fighter as well.

"Okay," I said, hitting the computer. "Let's see what we got." I googled "Names beginning with C that mean warrior."

And you know what? A ton of them popped up. Google is a godsend!

"Cade, Cadall, Caddock . . ." I began. "Caydman, Carney, Cadfer!"

Cory shook his head. "Nope, not feelin' it."

So I pressed on: "Carnel? Conlin? Charlton? Chevrolet?"

"Okay." Cory chuckled. "You are just making these up."

"I swear . . . they're right here! Along with Coil, Ciril, and Currin."

Then one name leaped out at me: "Cree. What about Cree?"

We mulled it over. It was originally Native Canadian (the Cree were great warriors and travelers), and it had a nice ring to it. The middle name just had to flow. So we decided on Cree Taylor . . . although Cayton Tristan was a close second.

Tamera loved the name from the start, but my mom wasn't so enthused: "Cree? What kind of name is that?" I assured her it was a great one, and I also loved that it meant "he believes" in Spanish. Besides, it was too late to change our minds. Cree Taylor it was!

Whether your main concern is honoring a family tradition or making sure that the name you choose for your child doesn't rhyme with anything particularly awful, my advice to you on baby naming is this: You should be able to name your child whatever you want. In retrospect, I would recommend not telling anyone that name until the baby is born. You'll certainly find out who to share what with as the time goes on.

12. **BREAST-FEEDING.** To nurse or not to nurse. It ain't no-body's business but your own. I have friends who swear by it, and had their babies on the boob long after the kid was able to ask for it. I have other friends who were adamant that they wanted to use formula. I planned to nurse, and if friends asked me I told them. Just be warned that people have very strong opinions on the subject.

13. **YOUR NAUGHTY DREAM ABOUT HAVING A HOTTIE FOR DESSERT.** Yum. Pregnant women, thanks to their raging hormones, often dream about sex. I sure did. And I was horny 24/7, too. Poor Cory! I think you can share this info with your hubby (just tell him it was him you were dreaming about—not Boris Kodjoe), and maybe he'll indulge your fantasy. Close girlfriends—yeah, sure. Your dreams these days are probably more entertaining than an episode of *Sex and the City* . . .

14. **EVERY FOOD THAT MAKES YOU NAUSEATED.** There is nothing more unappetizing than a pregnant woman who looks at your lunch plate and declares, "If I ate that, I'd hurl." I hear ya—morning sickness is the worst (see chapter 3 for some tips on how to keep it down). Just the smell of some foods could send me running for a barf bag. But I tried not to sicken everyone else by discussing what made me whoops. I suggest you do the same.

15. **MATERNITY SEX POSITIONS.** *Kama Sutra*, look out . . . I got some moves you ain't never seen! Again, it's those crazy hormones that make your muscles stretch in ways you

never thought possible. And frankly, you have to get creative if you want to get down to business with your man by month eight. As much as you'd love to brag to your buds about your acrobatics in bed, it should remain between the sheets.

CHAPTER 3

Barfing, Belching, and Hair Down There

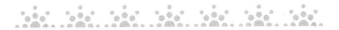

I know there are some women who look
incredibly beautiful when they're pregnant
and glow from head to toe. (Thank you,
Halle Berry, for showing up the rest of us.)
Not this woman. At best, I manage to stifle
a thunderous burp when I am eating in
public and make it to the ladies' room
before I hurl. I had no idea my body could
do some of the things it's been doing. I
thought only guys could be this gross.

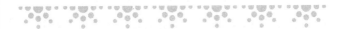

I can't say I wasn't warned. Friends told me their bodies behaved bizarrely during pregnancy. But I assumed most of it was manageable. So you got a little gassy and queasy from time to time—that comes with the territory, right? They say every woman is different and each experiences pregnancy in a unique way. That I buy. But I am convinced no one had all the crazy stuff that I did. This chapter isn't meant to freak you out; instead I hope it gives you some reassurance that no matter how bad you think you've got it . . . I can probably top that!

The Urge to Purge

If I had to sum up my pregnancy in one word, it would be *nausea*. Overwhelming, unrelenting, gut-wrenching nausea that came at the most inconvenient times. Like when I was having a lovely dinner out with friends, or in the middle of a romantic love scene on *The Game*. This nausea knew no boundaries and refused to be tamed! Trust me, I tried. I sucked on dozens of preggy pops, sipped cup after cup of ginger tea, accessorized with seasick bands (luckily, they come in so many pretty colors!). Nada. My OB kept reassuring me, "Oh, it'll stop in the second trimester . . . it'll stop in the third trimester." Guess what? It *never* stopped. I kept patiently waiting, and every time I thought I had conquered it, it would come a-knockin'.

Some doctors will tell you morning sickness comes from high levels of hormones, and others say genetics play a role (so if your mom escaped it, you might be lucky, too). I don't know what brought it on, but by week three of my pregnancy, I was in misery. This nausea—if you've yet to experience it—is not your average stomach-flu variety. It rolls over you like a tidal wave, with virtually no warning. Sometimes my mouth would get watery, and I could feel that "taste" creeping up the back of my throat. That was it: my only signal that I had mere seconds before whatever I had eaten made a repeat performance. I actually entertained the idea of carrying a barf bag with me (the kind they give you on airplanes), but I thought that would be a little too gross—not to mention too obvious while I was trying not to spill the beans (figuratively and literally!).

Shooting on a warehouse set in Atlanta made it even more complicated. I would have to leave the stage, usually dressed in heels and some sexy, tight dress, and race up a flight of stairs to reach the nearest bathroom. To make matters worse, the bathrooms were located right next to hair and makeup—so I would run the water and pray none of the stylists could hear me retching. Yes, I was a polite puker.

Oh, Baby!

Anything could trigger my nausea: watching a commercial for IHOP (the pancake syrup oozing was sickening!); catching a whiff of someone's perfume in an elevator; the sight, taste, or smell of onion, eggs, or chicken of any kind. But the thing that set me off the most? The scent of my man's body odor. My sense of smell was so heightened, I could detect the second Cory came through the door after working out at the gym. I would literally duck for cover and beg him to take a shower and Lysol the premises. Then there was his breath. I could eat garlic—and I would crave the taste. But if Cory ate some and I smelled it . . . it was all over. One night after we'd pigged out on a loaf of garlic bread, I couldn't sleep in the same bed with him. He brushed his teeth three times and used Scope, but I could still smell it. The Mama nose knows.

All this made me extremely pissed off at people who cheerfully told me they had no morning sickness. I figured there had to be some secret that no one was letting me in on. I even googled it: Miracle Cure for Morning Sickness. I tried all the suggestions:

- **GINGER CANDY AND TEA.** Supposedly, this remedy has been used for thousands of years. The herb is supposed to calm your stomach and even help headaches. While the taste cleaned my breath, it didn't do much for the rumbling in my stomach.
- **LEMONS.** You're supposed to sniff citrusy scents (or, even better, to suck lemons) to mask any noxious odors that might trigger your nausea. The lemon triggered mine.

- **SALTY CRACKERS.** An empty stomach can make nausea worse, so saltines keep you full between meals and hopefully less nauseous. They also make nasty crumbs in your bed (Cory will vouch for this).
- **ACUPRESSURE BANDS.** Those tight elastic bracelets with the little white studs that you wear if you get seasick or carsick. The theory is that these studs push on a pressure point that reduces nausea. For me, they worked sporadically; probably the pain of the plastic button digging into my wrist distracted me from my nausea.
- **BREATH MINTS, GUM, AND MOUTHWASH.** For me this was a no-go; a minty taste set me off on my pukey path. I had to find non-mint toothpaste, and chewing gum seemed to give me more gas. But women who complain of a tin taste in their mouths say minty flavor helps.
- **WATER.** When you're constantly throwing up, it's hard to stay hydrated—which is why I kept winding up in the hospital. Rinsing your mouth and sipping cold water is supposed to quell the queasies.

After much trial and error, what finally gave me some relief? Sourdough bread! I just discovered it one day. I had a piece and, lo and behold, my nausea subsided. I've heard of women eating bagels and pizza dough for similar reasons: thick bread acts like a sponge and absorbs stomach acid. Once I had my cure, there was no stopping me. I didn't even bother slicing it; I'd just tear into it with my teeth! I would wolf down several loaves a day and Cory would stare at me, wondering how and when the woman he loved had turned into a bread binger. I felt a little better—but I began gaining weight. Like, a lot of weight. Like fifty-seven pounds. Cree weighed seven pounds, twelve ounces—and I'm pretty sure most of the rest was sourdough.

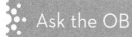

Ask the OB

Why do some women (like me) get morning sickness and some don't? It's not fair!

You're right, it's not fair, but about 70 to 85 percent of women suffer with some degree of morning sickness in their first trimester—you are not alone. Fewer than 10 percent experience nausea and vomiting beyond 20 weeks, and fewer than 3 percent of women suffer from the severe form called *hyperemesis gravidarum*. Morning sickness is currently believed to have evolved as a defense mechanism. The first trimester is the most critical for organ development in a fetus, and the time when the developing baby is most sensitive—and most at risk—to exposure to environmental chemicals or toxins. When exposed to the smell or taste of foods that might contain toxins dangerous to the fetus, women experience nausea to trigger avoidance of those potentially dangerous substances, even if they may be harmless to both of you. So, though you're miserable, just know it's your body's way of making sure baby is healthy!

To Pee or Not to Pee

I wish I could say things improved for me as I neared my due date. *Au contraire!* The bigger the baby got (and the bigger I got), the more the weight pressed on my bladder. Translation: Any sudden movement could cause me to spring a leak. Whenever I coughed, laughed, ran, sneezed, barfed, or burped, I was rewarded with what ranged from a trickle to a large stream down my legs. Cory considerately followed me around, putting towels under me. I wet myself wearing a beautiful teal silk dress during a magazine photo shoot. I tinkled at Tamera's bachelorette bash, just as the male stripper, dressed like a cop, started to bump and grind. Since you can't plug up the problem (though, trust me, I googled that, too!), I strongly recommend you familiarize yourself with the panty-liner aisle at the drugstore. Like a Girl Scout, you always want to be prepared. Trust me, the day will come when you will wee unexpectedly. My pee problem maxed out in my last month. Now I know what it must be like when you're ninety; I was constantly in a puddle. We were in the supermarket one day, and Cory took some Depends off the shelf and waved them at me: "You might wanna consider these." I cracked up . . . and promptly wet myself.

The Buzz on Fuzz

The werewolf dude in *Twilight* has got nothin' on me. During my pregnancy, hair suddenly sprouted up all over my body in places it had no business being! Like in a straight line from my belly button, pointing to my privates. My OB told me it was due to those lovely hormones again: they make facial and body hair grow faster, and this is called the *linea nigra* (literally, the "black line"). On most people, the *linea nigra* shows up as line of darker skin pigmentation; for me, it was that plus some newfound fur- riness. It tends to be more pronounced on darker skin, but luck- ily, mine was a light, sandy brown color. I figured it might come in handy in case Cory had trouble finding his way over my huge stomach during sex. I now had my own road map!

Girlfriends told me that hair can pop up anywhere: your boobs, back, stomach, arms. One pal confided that her nipples had suddenly sprung a few strays! I probably could have han- dled that; at least you can hide it under clothes. What freaked me out was the little 'stache growing on my upper lip. It was Cory who pointed it out (he doesn't notice the dirty dishes in the sink, but spies the peach fuzz on my face?). I raced to the bathroom mirror in a panic: yup, I needed a shave! The next day, I went and had it waxed—outta sight, outta mind. But I worried and wondered if I'd wake up one morning covered in fur. My doc reassured me that all the unwanted hair would be gone three to six months after I delivered. At the same time, some of my hair on my head (which felt thick, soft, and luxurious during pregnancy—a plus!) would fall out. Great. Now I had to worry about going bald, too.

The Gas You Pass

I liked to think of this as my baby's way of heralding his arrival with a thunderous trumpet blast. But truthfully, it's damn embarrassing to break wind. I would try to hold it in, but as my body took on the shape of a whoopee cushion, there was no stopping it. Of course, whenever I cut loose, I pretended it wasn't me. I would point the finger of blame (and fan the air) at anyone in the neighboring vicinity—my costars, my husband, the guy in front of me at the grocery checkout. Once again, those horrid hormones are to blame: they slow down the rate of food passing through your gastro tract. This gives some ladies constipation—and that goes hand in hand with gas. My advice: Eat more fiber, drink lots of water, and stay away from anything with bubbles in it (like soda). Some foods will just do it to you, for instance cabbage, cauliflower, Brussels sprouts, broccoli. And oh, those evil collard greens! But if it makes you feel better, the average pregnant woman farts about twenty times a day. So I figure I was right around that average. You should know, however, it's quality, not quantity, that counts!

My Best/Worst Fart Award goes to my appearance at a star-studded *Essence* magazine event. Jennifer Hudson, Jill Scott, Viola Davis—a virtual Who's Who of entertainers were there. I was seated at a luncheon table when suddenly I let one slip. I was praying no one heard or smelled my handiwork, and I could feel my cheeks (the ones on my face!) burn with embarrassment. I kept chattering away, pushing the food around on my plate, pretending I had no idea where that noxious odor was coming from. If anyone asked, it was the waiter.

The Burp Heard 'Round the Set

Whenever my sister and I were shooting our reality show, we were hooked up to microphones. In fact, after a while, I totally forgot they were there and just went about my business. One day, I forgot we were filming in front of an audience, and I let out this huge belch. It was amplified about a million times, and I practically blew out the mike guy's eardrums! He looked a little shocked, but then he cheered, "Yes! My kind of girl!"

Here's the funny thing I learned: Guys think it's great when a girl belches. Whenever I burped at the dinner table, in front of my male costars, even in Cory's face, I was met with the same reaction: "Awesome!" You can thank those good old pregnancy hormones (progesterone, in particular), which are slowing down digestion to allow more time for the nutrients from food to be absorbed into your bloodstream and passed to the baby. This makes you feel bloated and gassy, and I found the easiest way to relieve it was to belch—kinda like uncorking a bottle of champagne! I know it's gross and unladylike, but guys don't see it that way: I actually got standing ovations. And all this time I thought my talent was acting. Who knew?

Pregnancy Pimples

I was one of those teenagers you loved to hate—the one with beautiful, blemish-free skin. I prided myself on a perfect complexion. So you can imagine my horror when I started breaking out during my pregnancy. I am not talking just a little zit here or there, I am talking body acne! I had it all over my chest, and my face and hands were covered in scaly patches of eczema. The skin was actually peeling off my knuckles! I knew when I told my OB, she'd have some logical explanation (turns out hormones can make the glands in your skin get bigger and produce more oil). For my itchy skin, she suggested that I avoid drying situations (like hot showers or baths) and lather up with a heavy moisturizer or cocoa butter just after getting out of the water.

But I still felt like a "Before" picture in a commercial. The makeup artists on my shows were great with camouflage (see "Face Facts" on page 59), but I knew what was beneath those layers of pancake and powder. Where was that "pregnancy glow" that I was promised? Friends told me it could be a lot worse. Besides stretch marks, some women wind up with spidery veins, rashes, skin tags, and chloasma (a.k.a. the mask of pregnancy), where skin on the upper cheeks, forehead, and/or upper lip turns brown when exposed to the sun. The good news: All these freaky face and skin problems tend to disappear after delivery.

Face Facts

Plagued by pimples when you're preggers? Annoyed by itchy, sensitive skin? My makeup artist, Stacy Gibson, did a great job helping me clear up and cover up. Make sure you check with your OB before you use any over-the-counter acne medications. They can be absorbed through the skin and may be harmful to your baby.

- **Adjust your diet.** Foods that contain antioxidants—like salmon, dark green veggies, berries, cantaloupe, and extra-virgin olive oil—help fight off free radicals that can cause acne. Cutting back on sugar and white flour can do wonders for your skin (opt for whole grains instead). Also, unhealthy fats found in junk food and fried food can make acne flare up, so replace them with healthy fats like avocado and almonds.
- **Keep clean.** Wash your face morning and night with a mild, soap-free cleanser (I use Cetaphil, and Stacy recommends Dr. Bronner's castile soap). Make sure to rinse thoroughly, especially around your hairline and jaw, where pores tend to get clogged with excess oils. Don't scrub too hard, or you'll strip your skin of its natural moisture, which can cause your oil glands to work even harder to replace what you wiped away. Stacy told me not to use an exfoliant while I was pregnant, since skin is too sensitive for scrubs. And

don't squeeze or pick at pimples; they can become infected or, worse, leave a scar. Never go to sleep with your makeup on, and change your pillowcase every few days—so your face doesn't keep soaking up the same oil and bacteria.

- **Tone up.** Toner shrinks pores, gives your skin pH balance, and refreshes your skin—all good things for moms-to-be noticing unwanted changes in their skin. My makeup artist's DIY toner: Mix equal parts apple cider vinegar and coconut water. Apple cider vinegar has anti-inflammatory properties, and coconut water is high in trace minerals and extremely hydrating and, when used twice daily, can ease acne inflammation.

- **Depuff.** Along with the zits, you may find that your eyes suddenly look like you've done a few rounds in the boxing ring. Mine had dark circles under them all the time, and Stacy suggested I apply frozen dandelion-and-ginger tea bags to reduce the swelling. The natural tannins in the tea constrict the tiny capillaries below the skin surface, while dandelion root acts as a diuretic. Both ginger and dandelion have anti-inflammatory agents. Wet the tea bags, pop them in a ziplock, and throw them in the freezer. Place them underneath your eyes for five to ten minutes at a time. You can store them in the freezer until the next time you need them.

- **Hydrate.** My skin suddenly felt tight and itchy when I was pregnant. Stacy recommended that, along with water, I drink coconut water. It's high in potassium, chlorides, calcium, magnesium, and electrolytes—an instant "bath" for your skin.

- **Zap that zit!** Stacy swears that applying egg whites to a pimple will shrink it by morning. Dab some on with a Q-tip; the vitamin A in the whites is great for your skin, too!
- **Cover up.** Choose a concealer, foundation, and powder that match your skin tone. Apply a dime-size amount of foundation to the blemish, covering it and blending down, toward your chin. Next, dot on concealer with your finger and blend well. Finally, "set" with a pat of powder. You can dust off any excess powder. But a tip from my pro: Makeup applicators, like sponges, puffs, concealer applicator sticks, and brushes, can harbor bacteria. Instead, use clean fingertips, Q-tips, cotton balls, or disposable sponges and puffs, and remember to wash your makeup brushes often.

Well, Ain't This Swell?

One day in my last trimester, I woke up and my toes looked like those little pigs in a blanket they serve at cocktail parties. You should know I am a shoe girl (you saw the cover!), and to suddenly not fit into my fave size 7½ Report Signature heels was heartbreaking. My feet were swollen beyond recognition. They looked like two floppy balloons attached to my puffy ankles. I know, I know . . . it's par for the course. It even has a fancy name: edema. Knowing this didn't do much for me (I am sure you agree!). What did help immensely was splurging on a cute pair of Steve Madden sandals with a silver sequin strap—in a larger size. My feet breathed a tremendous sigh of relief the second I put them on. I wore them everywhere—even to my sister Tamera's wedding. I am just very lucky that I live in California, not, say, the frozen tundra. Although I hear mukluks are pretty comfy, too.

Nobody Nose the Trouble I've Seen

One day I was in my kitchen when blood started pouring down my face. I freaked. I had no idea why my nose was suddenly gushing. My first crazy-pregnant-lady thought was *brain tumor*. When I came back to my senses and called my OB, she said to take a deep breath (how could I? My nose was hemorrhaging!) and chill. Nosebleeds are very common for pregnant women, thanks to our increased blood supply. Basically, it ruptures fragile blood vessels in the nose, and there you have it: a gusher! I had never had a nosebleed before. Then again, I'd never been pregnant before.

Thirty percent of pregnant women also snore! It usually happens during the second and third trimesters, and experts think it comes from a combination of weight gain and increased blood flow, which causes blood vessels in your body to expand. As the vessels in your nose and throat enlarge, mucous membranes in the area begin to swell too, producing more mucus. So your breathing is obstructed, and your hubby is in for a symphony at night! Cory would tell me in the middle of the night to stop snoring, and I didn't believe him. I never snored before!

Oh, Baby!

My body was exhibiting so many bizarre new behaviors, I never knew what to expect next. I can happily report that I somehow sidestepped one particular pregnancy symptom: swelling down below. One pal shared with me the fact that her labia doubled in size and also popped up several purple varicose veins. Just picturing this made me nauseated (back to square one!), but slightly relieved. I know how easy it is to go all "Woe is me" when you're pregnant, to think no one else suffers this much or feels this lousy. I did. Most of us do. It also helps to know that most things that seem totally crazy-abnormal are perfectly normal during these nine months (okay, technically, ten, but who's counting? I'm trying to make you feel better here!). Any issue that arose, my doctor was there to help me deal with it—even the day I thought I was going blind.

Yes, you read correctly. My eyesight suddenly went fuzzy, and I found myself wearing my reading glasses all the time, even when I drove. Turns out, hormones decrease tear production, and your eyes can feel dry and irritated. The hormones can also cause fluid buildup in the eye (just like in my feet!) that can lead to vision changes. So there you have it. I wouldn't be blind, blemished, and barfing forever—just until I had my baby. A small price to pay, don't ya think?

Ask the OB

Why are my gums suddenly bleeding whenever I brush my teeth?

This is a very common problem for pregnant women. Pregnancy hormones can cause your gums to swell, become inflamed, and bleed more easily. Mild tenderness is normal, but if your gums are bright red, very sore, and bleed easily (your toothbrush has taken on a pink tinge, or you're spitting blood out when you rinse), you may have gingivitis, which is a mild and relatively harmless gum disease. But gingivitis can develop into the more serious condition called *periodontitis*, which is why good dental care is so important (research has also shown that periodontitis during pregnancy increases the risk of having a premature or low-birthweight baby). So, as long as you take extra care of your pearly whites and gums during pregnancy, you will avoid any complications.

Pregnancy Brain

And you thought it was just your body that suffers? I am living proof that your memory gets fried during pregnancy. I would forget phone numbers, where I put my cell phone (once in the fridge!), and whether or not I turned off the oven. I also left my keys in our front door all night—thank God we weren't vandalized! Sometimes it felt like I had peanut butter between my ears. Why couldn't I remember appointments? The next line in a scene? Those hormones were wreaking havoc again. Combined with the stress and the nausea, it's a wonder I knew my own name. And believe it or not, your brain-cell volume actually decreases during the third trimester. Yes, your brain shrinks! I am told by medical experts not to worry; it goes back to its original volume a few months after delivery. But in the meantime . . .

WRITE STUFF DOWN. Don't assume you will remember anything. I sure didn't. Jot dates on a calendar, e-mail or text yourself, or talk into a digital recorder. If you have to, scribble notes on your arm or leave yourself a voice-mail message. I memorized a mantra, "Take key out of car," and said it every time I parked, after the time I forgot and left the key in the ignition when I got out to go into the supermarket. Luckily, I remembered when I wasn't too far from the lot, and raced back to retrieve the key. After that I made an effort to carry around a yellow pad with me everywhere. Which was great . . . unless I forgot where I'd put it.

GET SOMEONE ELSE TO DO IT FOR YOU. I'm not kidding—delegate. I don't mean be a diva; ask politely. When you are juggling too many responsibilities, you are bound to let something slip through the cracks. Ask your friend/sis/mom/spouse if they can pick up your dry cleaning, drive you to an appointment, or pick up some groceries. I was pretty hesitant to burden people . . . until I was put on bed rest. At that point, stuck in my house all day, I was more than happy to ask favors of friends and family.

I even sent Tamera shopping for me. Since she's my twin, I figured she could hold up a dress, picture herself fatter in it, and choose a great look for my baby shower. I told my BFF, Jessica, I was hungry all the time, and she showed up with a huge container of homemade matzo ball soup. I didn't even know the woman could cook! It was the nicest thing any friend has ever done for me.

FIGURE OUT FUN WAYS TO REMEMBER THINGS. Try little rhymes, jingles, and visual clues. For example, one of my pregnant gal pals kept blanking on her new coworker's name. Though he told her several times, she just couldn't recall what to call him. She came up with a unique way to remind herself: Sea bass was her favorite fish (Chilean, to be exact)—she could eat a ton of it! So when he strolled by, she would think *sea bass ton*, and got his name instantly: Sebastian.

LAUGH AT YOURSELF. If you find your car keys in the freezer, cut yourself some slack. This fog will likely blow over a few weeks after you give birth. In the meantime, embrace your airheadedness. Someone asked me at a promotional event who my favorite actress was, and I totally blanked. I hemmed and hawed, and finally laughed and said, "There are too many for me to name!" I can always think of a million actresses I love, but in that moment . . . not a one.

Another time, Cory had just told me he was on the phone with Derrick, his stepfather.

"Who's Derrick?" I asked.

"You're kidding, right?" Cory replied.

"Give me a minute. It will come to me . . ." I racked my brain but, for the life of me, could not remember who Derrick was. I couldn't even picture his face.

Cory sighed: "Uh, my stepdad?"

"Oh, yeah!" I chuckled. "It was right on the tip of my tongue!" Frankly, my husband was lucky I didn't start calling him Cody or Mory . . .

Your friends and family may also realize that now is not the best time to be asking you to remember things for them. Case in point: My nine-month mark was a few days before Tamera's wedding, and I was supposed to be keeping her dress under lock and key. She knew me as the sister who was reliable to the point of list-making, but when I was pregnant, that all changed. I was busy remembering to pack my gown, my shoes, my purse, my jewelry, and my maternity Spanx to keep my new figure in place during her ceremony, when she called.

"You packed my dress, right?" she asked.

Gulp. I looked around the room. Where the heck did I put that big white silky thing?

"Oh, yeah. I um . . . I kind of forgot and left it in my car."

"You what?!" My sis was livid.

"I guess I forgot . . . you know, pregnancy brain?"

Yeah, she'd heard that one before. She dashed out of her house and drove over to mine, seizing the dress. I felt terrible, but it really wasn't my fault. My brain just wasn't working!

Ask the OB

With my pregnancy brain these days, I have
to write myself a note to take my prenatal
vitamins. Is it okay if I miss a few?

Prenatal vitamins are specially formulated multivitamins that
make up for any nutritional deficiencies in a mom-to-be's diet,
and let's face it, the average American diet may not be the most
nutritious. Prenatal vitamins contain various vitamins and minerals, and their folic acid, iron, and calcium content are especially
important. Folic acid can reduce the risk of severe spine and
brain abnormalities called *neural tube defects*. A baby with a
neural tube defect may have varying degrees of paralysis, incontinence, and sometimes mental retardation. Calcium taken during pregnancy and breast-feeding can help prevent your own
bones from thinning, as baby uses that mineral for its own bone
growth. Iron helps both the mother's and baby's blood carry
oxygen. While a daily vitamin supplement is no substitute for a
healthy diet, taking these supplements will ensure you are getting adequate levels of these minerals. They come in various
formulations, and sometimes it takes a little experimentation to
find one that doesn't leave you feeling queasy. Don't beat yourself up if you forget once, but these are important. Bottom line:
take them daily.

Blame It on the Hormones

Aside from all the freaky physical stuff going on, you can also chalk up the following to your changing body chemistry:

- **CLUMSINESS.** I became adept at tripping over my own two feet. My whole sense of balance and space was out of whack. I didn't seem to realize how large I was and would try to squeeze myself through cramped places. Or I'd wobble and fall over, or step on people's feet. Cory suggested I wear a sign: "Pregnant woman. Make way!" Your body is producing a hormone called *relaxin* (too bad I wasn't relaxin'!), which loosens the ligaments in your body, making you less stable and more prone to injury. It's easy to overstretch or strain yourself, especially the joints in your pelvis, lower back, and knees. So take it easy and try not to lift heavy things.

- **TIDINESS.** Your pregnant pals may have warned you about the instinct to nest. I'm usually a very organized person, but I turned into a super neat freak in my third trimester. I wanted to rearrange all the kitchen cupboards, the fridge, my dresser drawers, do loads of laundry, or scrub the bathroom sink. My house has never been cleaner! Just be careful not to overdo it; you'll tire yourself out!

- **SPACINESS.** I was so busy thinking about my baby, I couldn't concentrate on anything else. So I would constantly space out during conversations and change the subject, driving Tamera up the wall—especially when we were supposed to be talking about her wedding. If you find yourself caught not knowing what's going on, pause, take a moment to collect your thoughts, and ask someone to remind you, if you have to. Try to focus on the moment you're in—not on the million tasks you have to tackle.

The First Time I Felt the Baby Kick

With all the nonsense going on, your body expanding and your brain literally shrinking, it can be really easy to get overwhelmed with what's going on with your body. But then something wonderful happens inside you that makes you realize what it's all for.

I will never forget it: I was in my second trimester, watching *A Baby Story* on TV, and something in my belly did a little flip-flop. It tickled and I jumped. What the heck is that? It felt kind of like a butterfly kiss on the inside, or popcorn popping.

I wondered, was it indigestion (God knows I was gassy!)? *Flutter flutter flutter.* No, there was definitely something moving in there and it had rhythm! Hello, in there! Are you saying, "Hi, Mama?" Are you doin' the cha-cha?

I was so excited I ran to tell Cory, and he wanted to feel it for himself. He tried his best to get the baby to demonstrate his field kick. "You in there?" he shouted into my belly button. Amazingly, Daddy's booming voice actually calmed Cree down. But anytime I ate—especially something sweet or spicy—he responded with a little tap dance in my tummy. It was pretty amazing, feeling life growing inside me for the first time. It made it very real for me. Of course, then I worried: Is he moving too much? Too little? Why haven't I felt him move in the last five minutes? Dr. Kumetz encouraged me to calm down—sometimes Cree was actually sleeping!

Take a moment to enjoy those little flutters. Why? Because after you deliver, you'll lie awake at night missing them. It was the first connection I had with my son—our own little Baby–Mama Morse code.

CHAPTER 4

If I Want Your Opinion, I'll Ask for It

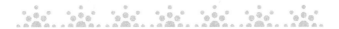

Everyone is telling me what I should do.
There is a contingent that tells me I must
have a natural birth with no drugs. These
people clearly want to see me suffer. I
think I have heard it all: hypnobirthing,
midwives, doulas, underwater births. A
friend of mine offered to give me a lesson
in vagina-stretching exercises so I could
"push that puppy out easier." Hello? Keep
your hands to yourself! Whose advice
should I take? The more I hear, the
more anxious I'm getting.

*T*here is no shortage of people who will tell you without a doubt that you are (a) doing everything wrong and (b) in need of serious redirection. I got it from all sides: friends, family, colleagues, critics, even the lady in the fast-food take-out window. Before I even knew I had to have a C-section, one friend told me I simply must insist on one: "It's so much more convenient! You can make an appointment, just like you'd book a blow-out at the salon!"

I was constantly biting my tongue and resisting the urge to tell well-meaning women to take their advice and stick it where the sun don't shine. But I am a lady. So instead I smiled, gritted my teeth, and tried not to think about the Big Day, which was getting scarier and scarier to consider.

Thanks, but No Thanks . . .

I know they meant well (at least, that's what they said), but the last thing I wanted was opinions from anyone other than my doctor. Want my advice (not really?) on the subject? Nod as if you are listening to every word and taking it in. Then do whatever you please—it's your body, your baby, your prerogative! Be on the lookout for these unauthorized infant instructors.

Your next-door neighbor with four-plus kids. This chick assumes she's got the whole birthing thing down. She's done it four times already and has another on the way, so that makes her a pro. I'll give you bonus points for being pregnant that many times—frankly, you deserve a medal of courage! Practice makes perfect, I always say. But just because listening to Mozart made your contractions easier does not mean it will work for me. Frankly, I am more of a hip-hop kind of girl. Each pregnancy is different, each woman is different, and each person's pain threshold is different. I am so happy to hear you pushed out a ten-pound baby with no drugs. If it were me, I'd want to be knocked out with a sledgehammer.

HOW TO HANDLE IT: Ooh and ahh at her amazing superhuman ability to deliver a new life into this world over and over and over again (is your uterus made out of rubber?). Give her a pat on the back, a round of applause, a nod in your book. Whatever it takes to make her go back to her brood and leave you alone.

The stranger on the street who asks to rub your belly. Yeah, my tummy is out there, big as a beach ball, for the whole wide world to see. But that does not mean I want you getting all touchy-feely on me! I am convinced some people think it's sweet and kind to pat a pregnant lady—or maybe lucky (yeah, I do kind of look like a Buddha). Not to worry, I am not lacking in attention or affection. What I need is for you to *step away from the stomach* and keep your hands where I can see them. I do not like being petted by strangers.

HOW TO HANDLE IT: Tempting as it is to go all Jackie Chan on this type, you're better off handling the situation with a little humor: "Well, you can look . . . but you can't touch!" or "If you rub mine, then I'll rub yours." If that doesn't work, I give you permission to say, "Crazy pregnant lady, high on hormones . . . touch me and lose a limb!"

Your hypochondriac coworker. Oh yeah, she is going to share every grisly, graphic detail of her hellish delivery with you. The blood. The gore. The forty-two hours of excruciating labor. The idiot hospital nurse who gave her the wrong meds. As if you weren't anxious enough—is she trying to push you over the edge? Suppress the urge to stuff a sock in her mouth. She's merely trying to bond with you. She thinks pregnancy is a sisterhood of suffering.

HOW TO HANDLE IT: Interrupt her politely and say, "I'm so sorry. I'm really nervous about my delivery, and I just can't listen to other people's scary stories. Maybe you should get in touch with someone who directs horror films!"

Your mom or mother-in-law who knows it all. Mother always knows best—at least the best way to drive you up a wall. You know that no matter how you respond, there is no winning.

HOW TO HANDLE IT: Even if you think she has no business minding your business, and you disagree 100 percent with what she is saying, don't take the bait. A grandma-to-be is not a woman to be messed with. Her emotions are running high and she is trying to assert her authority. Keep it simple and announce where you stand: "Thank you for your advice, but this is the way I prefer to do it." If she insists it worked for her, reiterate: "I'm sure it did, but I'm going to do it this way." If that's not getting through, you can always beg off and blame it on the hubby: "I'll have to discuss that with Cory!" If none of the above works, remember that arguing back will only make her more defensive and persistent. Instead, put on your best poker face. Cross your arms over your tummy (this is body language for "back off, it's my baby!") and look her straight in the eye. Do not flinch. She can smell fear. Then politely say, "Thank you for your concern. I appreciate it," and end the conversation before it gets ugly.

Above all, do not let anyone make you doubt yourself or your decisions. Yes, others might have more experience or knowledge, but you have to trust yourself and your instincts.

Ask the OB

Today at lunch my friend steered me away from my favorite *maki* roll and suggested I go with the chicken teriyaki, for my baby's sake. Are there things you can't eat when you're pregnant? Sushi? Smelly cheese?

I recommend avoiding any raw or undercooked meat or fish when you are pregnant. There are parasites and bacteria that can contaminate undercooked food, and although the chances of getting an infection from eating sushi or a rare steak are slim, the consequences are severe enough that you wouldn't want to take the risk.

Deli meat (turkey, pastrami, etc.), refrigerated smoked seafood (lox), and pâté have been known to harbor listeria, which can cause miscarriage and should be avoided. Listeria has the ability to cross the placenta and may infect the baby. Make sure to avoid refrigerated smoked seafood, and reheat any deli meat until it is steaming before consuming it.

Some fish contain very high levels of mercury and should be avoided. Mercury has been linked to developmental delays and brain damage. Among the fish that should be completely avoided are shark, swordfish, king mackerel, and tilefish. Canned tuna generally has a lower amount of mercury than other tuna, but should be eaten only in moderation. A good resource for fish-consumption guidelines is the Natural Resources Defense Council (NRDC) website: www.nrdc.org.

You can eat some cheeses when you're pregnant, and cheese is one of the good sources of calcium. However, some cheeses are not safe to eat. Soft, mold-ripened cheeses, such as Brie, chèvre, and Camembert; many of the blue cheeses, such as Gorgonzola and Stilton; and soft, unpasteurized cheeses, including goat's and sheep's cheeses, should be avoided. Even if they are pasteurized, they are more moist and less acidic than other, hard cheese varieties and provide the ideal environment for listeria to grow.

Where to Go for Info

I would highly recommend that your doctor be your go-to reference on all things pregnancy. But that still didn't stop me from opinion shopping, especially on the Internet. When Dr. Kumetz confirmed my baby was in breech, and advised me to consider a procedure to turn him, I went home and googled and got a ton of info that helped me make my decision. There are many good websites out there, chock-full of information that will come in handy. Here are a few of my faves.

Oh, Baby!

USE	WEBSITE	DESCRIPTION
To double-check on that thing your doctor told you about:	americanpregnancy .org	The national health organization covers everything from the medical side of your pregnancy, week by week, to info on prenatal tests and meds your OB might prescribe. A little clinical, but lots of good info.
If you want help creating your birth plan:	babycenter.com	They have all sorts of tools and calendars to help you track how things are going, and even tips on how reflexology can curb morning sickness—sign me up!
For more advice than you will ever know what to do with:	parents.com	Created by the editors of *Parents* magazine. This site's "Ask Parents" section quotes numerous experts and new moms, on topics ranging from fetal development to how to make baby food from scratch. I also like the blogs by real moms discussing real issues.
To find out what's going on this week in your pregnancy:	parenting.com	*Parenting* magazine's site lets you check in every week to read what's going on with your baby, your body, and a mom-to-mom observation. There are also cheap nursery ideas and a really funny page called "Show Dad How."
For maternity fashion trends:	celebritybabies. people.com	My guilty pleasure! I loved to see what trends were in for baby and me, and which celebs were expecting at the same time as me.

USE	WEBSITE	DESCRIPTION
When you're looking for some mommy gossip:	lilsugar.com	This site mixes gossip with shopping—my two favorite things. I admit it did make me a little envious to see how amazing Beyoncé looked with a bump—in a bikini... You go, girl!

What's Up, Doc?

I was very lucky to have such a close, personal relationship with my OB. Sometimes you are seeing a large practice, and a different doctor every time (could you at least tell me your name before you put your hand up there?). You may prefer one doctor's bedside manner or recommendations. Or sometimes, you're faced with a surprising complication, and suddenly you doubt your doc's advice. As in all relationships, communication is key.

- Write down everything you want to talk about before your visit or test. Remember that pregnancy brain! Make sure the most important things go at the top of your list, so you get to them first. If you run out of time, ask if you can call later or schedule another appointment. Make sure every question you have gets answered, and that you are clear on your doctor's response.
- Ask questions right away if you don't like the advice you are getting. Have your doctor draw you a diagram, pre-

sent research, even give you a referral for a second opinion. Don't be embarrassed to ask for one; he won't be
insulted. Express your concerns and hesitation and let
your doc do his best to reassure you. Have him outline
the risks involved in any procedure and what the pro-
spective results are. Sometimes the benefit (like an amnio
or genetic testing) can outweigh the risk.

• Spill your secrets. No matter how embarrassing the subject or question, I promise you that your doc has heard
it before. Sex during pregnancy, incontinence, strange
body odor . . . she can put your mind at ease if you speak
up. As you can see from my "Ask the OB" boxes, I did
not hold anything back! You should also share your family history, any past health issues—any conditions at all.
The doctor can do her best only if she knows everything
about you. Let her decide if it's important or not.

Ask the OB

Do doctors ever make mistakes when
they tell you the baby's sex?

The reliability of ultrasound to determine the baby's sex depends on several factors, including the age, size, and position of
the baby, the amount of amniotic fluid present, the thickness of
the mother's abdominal wall, the equipment used, the experience of the sonogram technician, and the cooperation of the

baby (sometimes they cross their legs so we can't get a good look!). The accuracy for determining fetal sex during the second-trimester sono (18 to 22 weeks) ranges from 95 to 99.5 percent—so you can be *pretty* sure. If not, you can schedule another sono to check again.

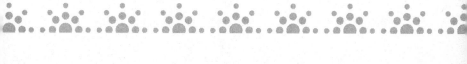

CHAPTER 5

Gimme, Gimme

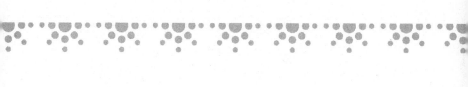

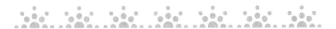

It happened in the middle of the night again. I woke up with a burning desire to eat a whole bag of crunchy onion rings. I've actually been dreaming about that yellow bag and see the neon-green letters dancing before me: FUNYUNS! FUNYUNS! FUNYUNS! You've probably heard the old wives' tales about pregnant women craving pickles and ice cream. Frankly, that never appealed to me. But Thai food at two a.m.? Pickled garlic? Fiery Cheetos? Now you're talking!

*D*espite the fact that I was constantly queasy, I still had powerful cravings and I was hungry often. I knew I had to eat to nourish the baby, so if there was a plate in front of me, I scarfed down whatever was on it (and then some).

At one point, Funyuns became all I could think about. Nothing would satisfy me until I had a mouthful of that delectable snack. I was prepared. I stocked my pantry with dozens of bags. Then, one night in the wee hours of the morning, another craving whispered in my ear. So I whispered in Cory's.

"Honey?" I said, rousing him from a deep sleep. "I need something."

Cory jumped up, thinking something was wrong. "Wuh? Huh? What do you need?"

"McDonald's french fries." It was all I could think of, a mountain of salty, greasy goodness! If I didn't get it, I would die.

"Really?" Cory groaned.

"Really," I insisted. "I have to have them. *Now*."

Bless his heart, he went to the Micky D's drive-thru and brought me home an extra-large box—which I polished off in bed with a huge smile on my face.

No one really knows for sure why you crave what you crave; it's shifting pregnancy hormones at work, and a heightened sense of smell and taste that make certain foods irresistible. And it can change from pregnancy to pregnancy. One friend of mine would eat entire tubs of Duncan Hines frosting when she was pregnant with her daughter, but with Baby Two, she wanted only Triscuits topped with peanut butter. Sweet treats now sickened her (and yes, she was carrying a boy!). Cravings can also change from day to day (hence my Funyuns-to-fries conversion). When I was first pregnant, I loved fiery Cheetos. By the end of my first trimester, I never craved them anymore. And after you deliver, you may even find your favorite foods now turn you off. Sadly, I don't think I could look at a Funyun for a long, long time . . .

Some experts believe that cravings are actually your body's signal for the nutrients it needs to feed the growing fetus (if that's the case, Cree should have been born with onion breath!). Thanks to sourdough bread and onion rings, I was gaining weight at an alarming rate. My doc sat me down at about five months for a warning: Putting on too many pounds during pregnancy increases the risk of gestational diabetes and unhealthy blood pressure. Gulp.

"I can't help it," I told her. "The Funyuns . . . they call to me."

The trick she shared with me is to honor your cravings . . . but be smart about it. For example, if all you can think about is a large pizza with the works, make yourself a whole-grain English muffin topped with tomato and melted low-fat mozzarella. You'll trick your taste buds without packing on the pounds.

You Say Potato Chip, I Say Popcorn

The following food swaps will satisfy you without expanding your waistline—you have the baby doing that already!

IF YOU CRAVE...	OPT FOR	BENEFITS
Ben & Jerry's Cherry Garcia	Nonfat chocolate frozen yogurt	It will satisfy your craving for cold and creamy and save you about 75 calories per serving. Top with some fresh or frozen cherries, which are rich in antioxidants.
A box of Godiva	Nonfat chocolate syrup drizzled on your fave fresh fruit	These chocolate-covered strawberries are so decadent—and have only about 35 calories each. Plus, the fruit is packed with vitamins and fiber.
A jar of Jelly Bellys	Chewy dried fruits (apricots, mango, raisins, and cranberries)	A handful of these (about 1/3 cup) will satisfy your sweet tooth, plus you can sprinkle them on cereal and salads and boost your fiber (translation: They'll keep you full).

IF YOU CRAVE . . .	OPT FOR	BENEFITS
A can of Pringles	Air-popped popcorn	If the taste of salt is seducing you, opt for this treat sprinkled with a seasoning blend, and you can have 3 cups for less than 100 calories.
A pitcher of lemonade	Half a grapefruit	This fresh snack will end your quest for tart, with only 32 calories. It's also rich in vitamins A and C, potassium, folate, iron, and calcium.

A Healthy Pregnancy Eating Plan

Eating well isn't just about keeping those extra pounds off to keep you healthy. It's not only you who are what you eat . . . your baby is, too! The food you consume is actually helping to build all your baby's organs. My nutrition consultant and chef Melissa Larsen has taught me so much! She says it's a good idea to avoid processed foods, sugars (including fruit juice), wheat, and glutens if you want to stay strong and healthy during your pregnancy. I did a great job sticking to this plan until the last trimester—that's when my cravings kicked in and I stopped following it religiously. I have also found it to be a great diet to follow when you're trying to shed your baby weight.

Throughout the day, make sure you are eating frequent small meals and snacks that are rich in nutrients. This plan is based

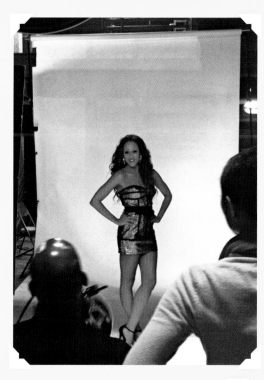

*Moments from the
first trimester,
when I knew and
no one else knew.*

You can see it on my face!

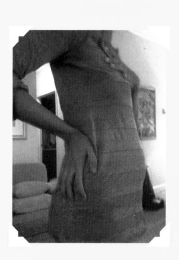

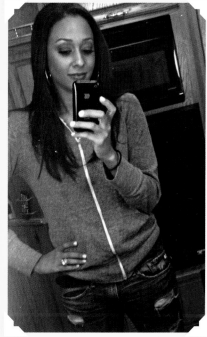

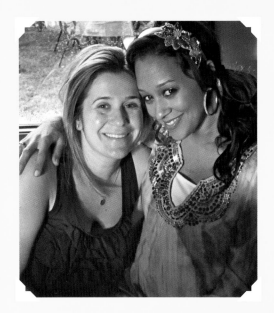

Soon there was no hiding my bump!

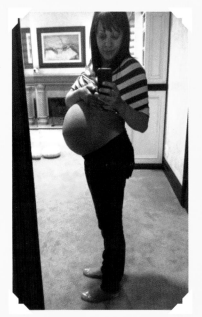

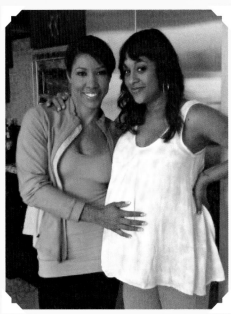

Top left, with Jessica; bottom right, with Jeanette Jenkins, my trainer.

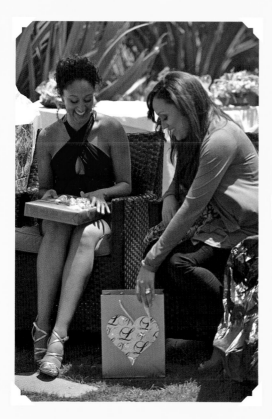

Flauntin' it in my favorite flats and cardigans, at home and at Tamera's bridal shower.

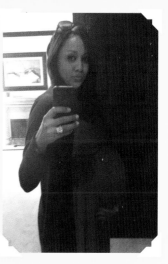

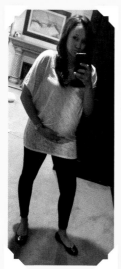

With friends at Essence's Black Women in Hollywood luncheon.

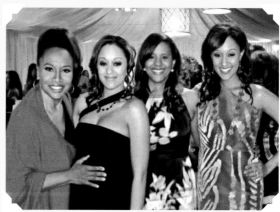

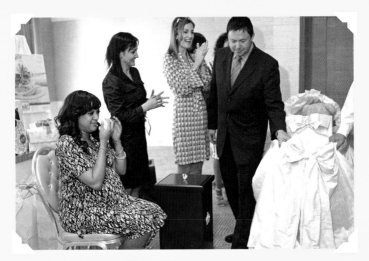

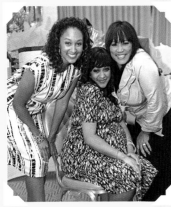

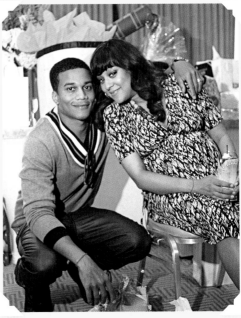

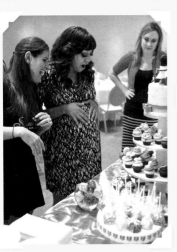

My baby shower!

With Cory, friends, and family—including my TV mom Jackée. I was eyeing those cake pops, and was overwhelmed by the outpouring of love.

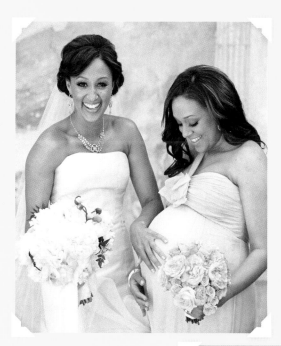

*Ready to pop
during Tamera's
wedding weekend.*

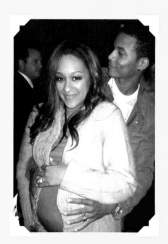

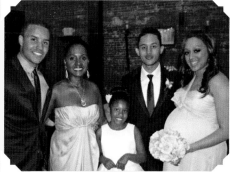

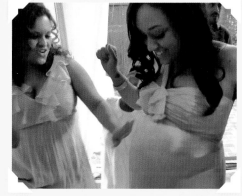

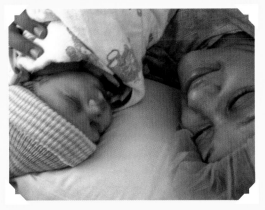

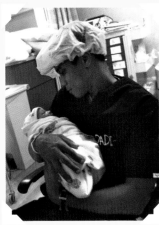

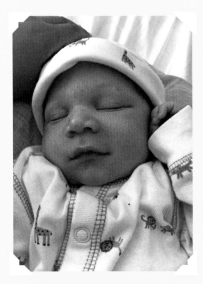

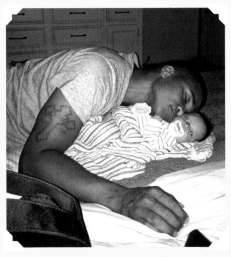

The big day—I have never
seen anything so beautiful
and perfect in my life.

Back at work, on the set of
The Game *with my little man.*

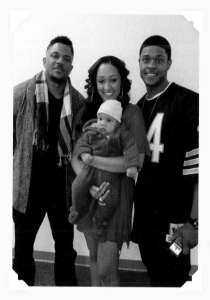

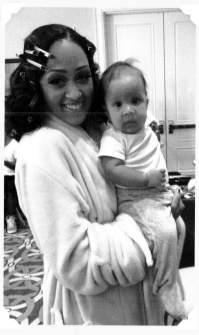

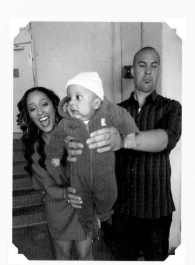

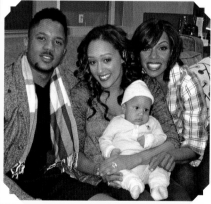

*Top left, with Hosea Chanchez (left)
and Pooch Hall (right); bottom left,
with Coby Bell; bottom right, with
Hosea Chanchez and Wendy Raquel.*

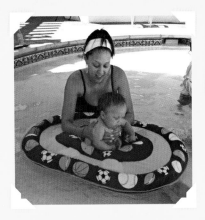

Cree's milestones:
first swimming lesson,
time on a plane,
reading together,
and first Halloween!

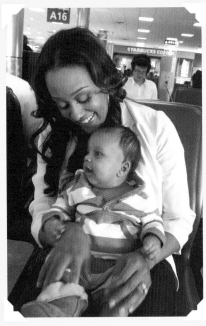

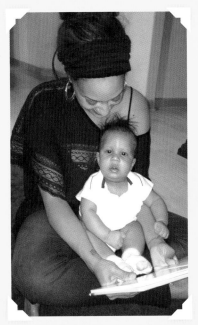

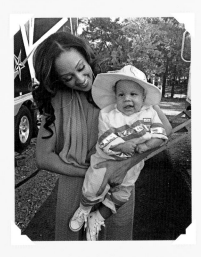

on the principles of the Body Ecology Diet (BED), which always fills me with energy and keeps me mean and lean! The BED recommends that your meals be 80 percent vegetables (prefer-ably organic) and 20 percent protein or grain (and advises that all animal proteins be eaten before two p.m., as it is easier on the digestive system).

A Menu for
Mamas in the Making

Morning Wake-up Drink

Start the day by alkalinizing the body for maximum strength and energy. Drink one glassful in the morning, and drink more glasses throughout the day, if desired. You can make "lemonade" by adding a few drops or more of stevia.

Juice of 1/2 lemon squeezed into a glass of room-temperature purified water

Breakfast

Think protein, veggies, and whole grains to give you long-lasting energy. I would load up on eggs and quinoa, and that recharged my batteries.

¾ cup quinoa flakes or gluten-free oatmeal served with stevia, cinnamon, and almond milk

or

2-egg omelet, with 2 cups of vegetables of your choice

or

2 soft-scrambled eggs, 2 cups of spinach, zucchini, and garlic

1 slice turkey bacon

and

1 tablespoon cultured vegetables* (gradually increase to ½ cup)

*Cultured vegetables are soft, delicious, and somewhat pickled through a fermentation process that increases the friendly bacteria naturally present. They are chock-full of probiotics and digestive enzymes (so a pregnant woman's system will be armed to support the immune system and digestion) and can be found at your local health food store.

Lunch

Protein plus salad will keep you full and will calm cravings. Although my cravings were tough to tame, I knew that eating these lunch dishes gave me great nutrients and fiber and satisfied my hunger. I was working fourteen-hour days, so I needed to stay full.

Grilled chicken and veggies on a bed of greens

or

Lamb chops and mixed greens sauté

or

Turkey Lettuce Wraps with Herb Vinaigrette (see recipe, p. 95)

and

1 tablespoon cultured veggies (gradually increase to 1/2 cup)

Turkey Lettuce Wraps with Herb Vinaigrette

Makes 2-3 servings

Large romaine leaves	1/2 cup grated carrot
1 pound cooked turkey breast,	1/2 cup fresh basil (whole leaves,
shredded or cubed	or chopped to a fine shred)
1/2 cucumber, chopped	

HERB VINAIGRETTE

1/2 cup grapeseed oil vegannaise	Juice of 1/2 lemon
(vegan mayonnaise)	1 teaspoon oregano or thyme

Mix well, and add water to create desired consistency. Fill each romaine leaf with turkey, veggies, and basil. Top with vinaigrette, and roll ends of each lettuce leaf together.

Dinner

One thing I have learned from this diet is that you can have a delicious, satisfying meal with no meat. (Or go for a tasty seasoned fish that's rich in omega-3.)

Stuffed Red and Yellow Bell Peppers (see recipe, p. 97)

or

**Cod Infused with Ginger, Cilantro, and Chives
(see recipe, p. 98)**

or

Salmon Dijon (see recipe, p. 98)

Stuffed Red and Yellow Bell Peppers

Makes 2 servings

2 bell peppers, 1 red and 1 yellow	2 large garlic cloves, crushed
(cut tops off, remove seeds,	1/8 teaspoon grated ginger
and set aside)	1 1/4 cups cooked quinoa
1/2 cup diced yellow and red	3/4 cup cooked millet
bell peppers (use tops you	1 tablespoon grapeseed or
removed)	olive oil, plus more to oil the
1/2 small yellow onion, chopped	baking dish
1/4 cup diced zucchini	1 1/4 teaspoons spicy herb
1 cup shredded cabbage	seasoning (I prefer Trocomare)

Preheat the oven to 375°F. Heat 1 tablespoon grapeseed or olive oil in a large skillet. Sauté all vegetables (except peppers to be stuffed) on medium heat for 4 minutes, stirring occasionally. Add quinoa and millet and mix. Pack filling into peppers. Oil a Pyrex dish with the grapeseed or olive oil and place the peppers in it. Cover and bake for 45 minutes.

Cod Infused with Ginger, Cilantro, and Chives

Makes 2 servings

2 skinless 6-ounce pieces of cod	1 tablespoon finely chopped
1 tablespoon grated ginger	cilantro and chives
	1 tablespoon wheat-free tamari

Preheat the oven to 375°F. Wash cod well and place in a Pyrex dish filled with 1/2 inch water. Spread ginger over the cod. Cover and bake for 20 to 25 minutes. After cooking, add cilantro and chives, and top with tamari.

Salmon Dijon

Makes 2 servings

2 skinless 6-ounce pieces of wild salmon	2 tablespoons crushed garlic
	2 tablespoons grated ginger

DIJON SAUCE

2 teaspoons Dijon mustard	2 teaspoons water
2 teaspoons wheat-free tamari	2 drops stevia

Preheat the over to 375°F. Wash salmon well and place in a Pyrex dish filled with 1/2 inch water. Spread garlic and ginger on salmon. Combine ingredients for Dijon Sauce, mixing well, pour over salmon, and cover. Bake for 20 to 25 minutes.

What Mama Wants, Mama Eats

Even with a filling, healthy diet, those cravings tend to kick in and they must be tamed. I used to get hungry in the middle of the night. Melissa told me to keep some almonds by my bed, but she also whipped me up some special treats. The great thing about these snacks is that they don't just taste good, they're also good for you and your baby. Don't forget to share!

Green Smoothie

Makes 4 servings

1 avocado	1 tablespoon herb of choice—
1 Granny Smith apple	cilantro, basil, parsley—or
4 ribs celery	1/2 teaspoon ginger
1 medium cucumber	1 teaspoon lemon juice
2 kale leaves, stems removed	4 cups purified water
1 cup chopped romaine leaves	

Chop veggies and fruit small. Add all ingredients to a blender or food processor, and blend until smooth.

These were great mid-morning, when I could hardly wait until lunch!

Tia's Chocolate Chip Cookies

Makes 12 cookies

2 cups almond meal	1 tablespoon nonalcoholic vanilla
1/2 cup whole-grain flour	extract
1/4 teaspoon sea salt	1/2 cup applesauce
1/4 teaspoon baking soda	1 cup grain-sweetened
1/2 cup plus 2 tablespoons cultured	chocolate chips
butter or ghee, melted	

Preheat the oven to 350°F. Combine all dry ingredients in a large bowl. Mix in wet ingredients and fold in chips. Form the cookie dough into 1 1/2-inch balls and press onto a pan lined with parchment paper. Bake for 10 minutes. Let cool and serve.

These are so delicious,
I used to dream about them!

Bliss Balls

Makes 12 balls

1 cup raw almond butter	¹/₂ teaspoon stevia
¹/₂ cup carob powder	¹/₄ teaspoon sea salt
¹/₄ cup water	Handful of almonds, finely
1 teaspoon nonalcoholic vanilla	chopped
extract	

Combine all ingredients except almonds, and mix well. Form into bite-size balls. Coat with chopped almonds. Store in an airtight container in the refrigerator.

Great to pack for a midday work snack.

Ask the OB

Is it safe to exercise when you're pregnant?

You should always ask your doctor first before starting any exercise program. I would recommend, in the absence of any pregnancy complications, 30 minutes of moderate exercise per day on most, if not all, days of the week. Pregnancy hormones cause the joints of the body to relax. Exercise will help the supporting muscles protect your back, abdomen, and pelvic floor, and good body alignment will help prevent or lessen many of the discomforts of pregnancy. Exercising during pregnancy will also help you stay in shape for labor and delivery, and it will help prevent too much weight gain. Make sure you have a warm-up and cool-down period, and avoid exercises that cause you to strain and hold your breath. Also, stay away from exercises that put too much pressure on your lower back or have you lying flat on your back. Be sure to avoid high-contact sports, scuba diving, and anything that comes with a high risk of falling or abdominal injury, such as gymnastics or certain yoga poses. Stop exercising immediately if you experience any chest pain, shortness of breath, dizziness, vaginal bleeding or leakage of fluid, or regular contractions.

Keeping Fit

Long before I got pregnant, my trainer, Jeanette, taught me that fitness involves both body and mind. Using that philosophy, she got me into the best shape of my life for *The Game*. When I was pregnant, there were so many times I did not want to work out! It was great to have Jeanette there to push me to get my butt off the couch, do one more crunch, one more hip raise.

Once I hit my second trimester, found the sourdough, and started to pack on a few pounds, it was easy to feel that there was no point to my efforts to feel and look like a hot mama. "Sexiness is not defined by body size," Jeanette assured me. Here are some of her best tips, which kept me motivated and will keep you moving. A healthy mama means a healthy baby, and there's no better gift you can give yourself than starting an exercise routine. You'll love the way you look and feel, and that will translate tenfold to the rest of your life. Trust me.

Top 10 Tips to Stay Active During Pregnancy

1. **Pump up the volume.** Create a motivating playlist on your MP3 player. Research proves that music motivates you to move. Some of my favorite tunes that get me pumped up lately are Beyoncé and Jay-Z's "Crazy in

Love," Justin Timberlake's "SexyBack," and Natasha Bedingfield's "I Wanna Have Your Babies." Don't tell Cory about that last one.

2. **Join a support group.** Join a prenatal exercise class that meets once a week. Check your local health clubs and yoga studios for listings. Sharing the workout experience with other pregnant moms is motivating and creates an instant support group.

3. **Prioritize.** Schedule your workouts into your weekly schedule just like any important meeting. If your workout is scheduled, then there is a much higher likelihood that you will do it.

4. **Start your day with a morning workout.** Dedicate your first waking moments to you, your baby, and your health. As the day goes on, your schedule gets busier and you also get tired. Working out first thing in the morning will help you clear your mind, and circulate oxygen and endorphins through your body so you start your day feeling great.

5. **Seek professional help.** You go to a mechanic to maintain your car and a dentist to care for your teeth, so why not consider going to a certified personal trainer to help take care of your body? By hiring a trainer to meet with you once a week, you'll have someone to keep you on your toes and show you how to do the exercises correctly. Again, keep your doctor in the loop, and look for a trainer who specializes in pregnant clients.

6. **Energy creates more energy.** It's normal to not feel like working out sometimes, but that's probably when you need it the most. When you're feeling tired or stressed, even a fifteen-minute walk will send endorphins through your body and make you feel better. Think about how amazing you will feel when you are done with your workout, and get moving.

7. **Make it fun.** Just because you're expecting doesn't mean that you can't have a fun workout. You can still dance, cardio box, swim, hike—whatever you enjoy. Just make sure that you stay within your safety zones. This is not the time to try new exercises, but if you were already doing these types of workouts before you got pregnant, then you can keep doing them.

8. **Mix it up.** To make sure you don't get bored with your workouts and to help you stay motivated, make sure your weekly workout plan has a variety of different methods of training: cardio (walking, hiking, stationary bike, spinning, aqua fitness, dance, aerobics, cardio boxing); muscular strength and endurance (sculpting, ballet, traditional weight training); and flexibility (Pilates, yoga, stretching).

9. **Get inspired.** Post a picture up on your fridge or bulletin board that motivates you to stay active. Think of what inspires you: your favorite athlete or celebrity, or quotation or scripture; an active, healthy pregnant mom; a favorite dress or bathing suit you would like to wear after

your pregnancy; or a vacation spot that inspires you to work out.

10. **Be positive.** This is an often overlooked part of your health, but it's even more important when you're pregnant. Make the choice to look for the positive in every new challenge and experience that comes your way. If you react to life with negativity and stress, then you will be sending those stress hormones to your baby. A happy mommy makes a happy baby. If all else fails, laugh it off—tomorrow's a new day.

Ask the OB

When will I fit back into my clothes, and what will my body look like post-pregnancy?

Between the baby, the placenta, and the amniotic fluid, you typically leave the hospital about 10 to 15 pounds lighter than when you came in—which constitutes your initial weight loss. However, your belly bump won't be completely gone. Most new mommies still look about 5 months pregnant on the day they are discharged from the hospital. By 6 weeks postpartum, many women have lost about two-thirds of their pregnancy weight, assuming they gained the typical 25 to 35 pounds. Your goal for weight loss should be about 1 to 2 pounds per week.

If you developed stretch marks during your pregnancy, and most women do, the good news is they fade over time. The bad news is they don't go away completely. There are some creams that you can try, but don't expect miracles. Most don't offer very dramatic results. The good news about the linea nigra—the brown line many pregnant women get on their belly—is that it will disappear completely, usually within 6 months, though if you are nursing it may take a little longer.

One of the most significant post-pregnancy changes your body goes through is actually above your belly bump . . . your breasts. Most expecting mommies get bigger breasts while pregnant—and they get even bigger while nursing. But afterward, they will not remain bigger—just longer and a little flatter. While your breasts may regain some of their original shape, they rarely look exactly the same as they did before pregnancy. Your arms, on the other hand, will soon start to look leaner and stronger. You will be carrying your baby—a lot—and that usually leads to nicely toned biceps.

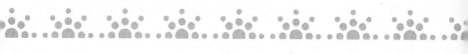

CHAPTER 6

Loco Emotions

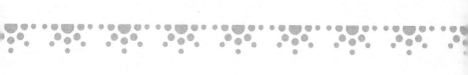

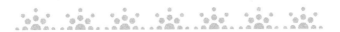

This morning, I totally lost it. Everything was irritating me: my pants wouldn't zip, I felt like throwing up (again!), and I was stressing over telling Tamera I wasn't up to attending her bachelorette weekend. I knew she was going to freak.

Noticing my nasty mood, Cory tried to be sympathetic: "Baby, I know it's uncomfortable . . ."

"Excuse me? You know it's uncomfortable? You know? How could you know? Are you pregnant? I don't think so!"

I was the one carrying this baby, puking my guts out, changing my diet, and going through daily hell. *I* had to undergo all the tests and the poking and prodding of my private parts—not Cory. In fact, *he* was the reason I was in this situation! When I looked at my man at that moment, all I could see was red. Cory tiptoed away, wondering when his mild-mannered, loving wife had turned into Attila the Mom.

I felt like I was at the mercy of my body: I was exhausted, queasy, and unable to think clearly. I had always prided myself on how much I could juggle. Now I felt like a big fat failure. I was letting people down—especially my sis before her wedding day—and there was nothing I could do about it. My mind said, "Go," but my body was screaming, "Stop!" I wasn't in control of my life anymore. At times I felt furious, while other moments I burst into tears. My emotions were on overdrive, and anything could set me off. I was like a ticking bomb with a very, *very* short fuse. Everything agitated me. I don't think Tamera and I have ever argued as much as when I was preggers. When we went to Sweet E's to taste cupcakes for my baby shower, I almost bit her head off when she ate my vanilla confetti cake pop.

"You don't take a pregnant woman's cupcake!" I screamed at her, wrestling the empty pop stick out of her hand.

"Geez," Tamera replied. "You are so hormonal!"

For the record: I hated when anyone told me I was hormonal. I knew I was hormonal; I did not need to be reminded. And if you didn't instantly sympathize with all my aches, pains, and agita, or rush to refill my cup of water, it was war. I resented anyone and everyone who wasn't in my too-tight shoes.

Ask the OB

Am I crazy ... or just pregnant?

You're not crazy! You have a lot going on, from a biological standpoint: Human chorionic gonadotropin, or hCG, rises in the first trimester, then dips and levels off around four months. Progesterone and estrogen increase throughout the nine months. These hormones can cause morning sickness and can also make you feel moody. Remember that pregnancy is as much an emotional journey as it is a physical one. Get lots of sleep, communicate what you need and want, and ask for help from friends and family if you're feeling overwhelmed. I promise you, you're not nuts! Almost every pregnant woman experiences these feelings at some point.

Baby Shower Cake Pops

Makes 12 pops

1 cup crumbled white cake; use your favorite recipe	Lollipop sticks
Sprinkles	16 ounces white chocolate candy, for coating
¼ cup vanilla frosting; use your favorite recipe	

In a large mixing bowl, rub the cake together with your fingers until it is all crumbs; mix some of the sprinkles in with the cake crumbs.

Mix the vanilla frosting in with the crumbs until the mixture can hold its own shape; use more frosting if needed.

Roll the mixture into 1-inch ball shapes with the palms of your hands. Place the balls on a cookie sheet lined with parchment paper. Put a lollipop stick into the top of each one, and then put in freezer for 30 minutes to 1 hour.

Melt the white chocolate in a microwave-safe bowl in 30-second intervals, stirring in between.

When your cake balls feel chilled (not frozen), dip them into the melted chocolate and, while the chocolate is still wet, add sprinkles and place back on the cookie sheet to set up. Repeat with remaining cake balls. If making ahead for a party, you can store in the fridge for up to five days. Eat and enjoy!

These Vanilla Confetti Cake Pops from Sweet E's are the perfect treat for a baby shower, and your guests will love them.

Feelin' Not So Groovy?

I know, I know: Some women coast through their pregnancies, feeling no mental anguish. The rest of us mere mortals are emotional basket cases. While every lady is different, it helps to know what you might be in for, given your wacky hormones and the normal stresses you have to deal with at each stage of *The Game*.

First Trimester

You're feeling ANXIOUS. No matter how prepared you think you are for this moment, reality slaps you in the face. Along with the joy of finding out you're expecting comes the worry: Is the timing right? Will we have enough money? Will my boss freak out? Do we have enough room? Will the baby be healthy? I felt like my mind was racing all the time, trying to process every what-if. I also began to doubt that I was ready to change my life so dramatically—and I was terrified of what labor and delivery would be like. In a nutshell: I have never felt so anxious in my life. It gets better, I promise.

Second Trimester

You're feeling LARGE. This is the time when most women start to show, so you're dealing with having to tell everyone, as well as the fact that nothing in your closet fits anymore. The weight gain made me depressed; I dreaded every time I had to go shopping (so not like me!) because it meant facing a full-length mirror. This is also the time you're coping with a ton of scary tests, such as amnio and other genetic tests to detect birth defects, and a glucose screening. With every sonogram, I got nervous that something would be wrong ("What's that thing between its legs?! Oh, yeah . . ."), and Dr. Kumetz had to calm me down. I cried all the time, and for no reason: I once started to sob when I was watching *Avatar*. I cried through that entire movie. Cory stared at me. "Tia, are you serious? Why are you hysterical?"

"It's just so beautiful," I wailed. "The trees! The lights! The blue people!"

Another time, I finished a workout and Cory teased me, "Honey, you stink." That was it. I broke down and bawled: "Oh my God, you told me I stink! That is so mean! How could you say that?"

Cory just laughed, which made me cry even more: "Why are you laughing at me? That's so awful!"

Third Trimester

You're feeling EXHAUSTED. The bigger my belly grew, the more tired I got. Think about it: I was dragging around an extra fifty pounds! The fatigue was frustrating and depressing: while all my sister's friends were having fun, drinking wine and partying on her wedding weekend, I was in bed, unable to pick my head up off the pillow. I constantly felt like a third wheel, a burden, a blimp. And as my due date drew close, I was also increasingly fed up. I just wanted this pregnancy to be over and the baby to be out! At the same time, I was petrified and having nightmares about my C-section. My OB assured me it's natural to be scared with your first pregnancy; you don't know what to expect. Even moms who have had two or three kids get nervous before the Big Day, because every delivery is different. OMG... what happens if I want to go through this again?

I even dragged Cory to an appointment with Dr. Kumetz so she could explain that my tirades and tantrums were just a combination of hormones and stress. I felt terrible that Cory had to get the brunt of it, but he lived with me. He was in the line of fire most of the time. I felt like no one was listening to me, and the only way for me to be heard was to stamp my feet and yell.

When I finally calmed down, I saw that I was overreacting and being unfair to the people I loved. Tamera and I were both going through huge moments in our lives, and I had to cut her some slack and try to understand how stressed she was, too. As for Cory, I realized how lucky I was to have him in my life. He's such a great guy, and I honestly don't know how he put up with me! Dr. Kumetz reminded me that he was going through a lot as well. He was probably nervous about being a dad and frustrated that he couldn't help me feel better. So he wasn't *purposely* trying to piss me off; he just didn't know what to say or do.

Oh, Baby!

It was like a lightbulb went on in my head: *Tia, it's not just about you.* I realized that Cory and I were in this together. I also realized that the things that were making me angry at him weren't all that important. Stuff like his dragging his feet when he got out of the car ("Will you hurry up?") or leaving the toothpaste cap off the tube ("Why do you have to be so sloppy?"). I apologized: "It was the hormones talking, not me."

"Yeah, I know," he replied, giving me a hug. "It's okay." Is this man amazing or what?

I promised to remember that we're a team—and Cory vowed to be patient and understand if occasionally (okay, maybe daily) I needed to vent and throw things. Stuff will come up between you: that's a given. Maybe you want to take a Lamaze class, and he thinks it's a waste of time. Or you want to puree all your own organic baby food, and he wants to buy jars at Costco. You both want the same things: a happy, healthy baby and an easy, safe delivery—and you want to be good parents. We moms-to-be (since we're the ones carrying around the bambino for nine months) tend to pull rank and get our way with most things. Give your hubby some consideration; hear him out. Let him air his concerns without fear of being shot down. He cares—give him credit for that. If he's got a strong opinion one way or the other, it means he's freaking out just like you are, worrying about all the possible and probable outcomes of this pregnancy. Is it honestly such a big deal if he prefers not to go to every birthing class, and your sis subs for him? I say choose your battles wisely.

Case in point: Cory was big on having me breast-feed. He did his homework; he believed that breast milk was the healthiest choice for our baby. That's fine; I'm all for it. But I worried how I'd be able to nurse and work at the same time.

"I'm okay if we have to supplement with formula now and then," I told him.

Cory wasn't. "Can't you just pump faster?"

I bristled. "Seriously? Do I look like a mama cow? I'll pump as fast as I can, but it takes time. And sometimes the milk just doesn't cooperate." He assumed each breast had a quart on hand at a minute's notice.

We argued over this for quite some time, until finally Cory realized Mama Knows Best.

We Can Work It Out

Even though my hubby was a prince during my pregnancy, we still had our share of spats. We were both nervous and facing a *major* change in our life as a couple. Cory, to his credit, didn't blow his top and tried to let me have my way . . . most of the time. But as we got further along into the pregnancy, we both got more and more stressed. It was virtually impossible to always see eye to eye on everything. But we took a vow in our marriage: Never go to bed angry. This meant no matter how livid I was that he changed the channel on the remote while I was watching, we had to kiss and make up. By the morning, my pregnancy brain had pretty much erased the entire incident anyway.

If you're feuding, here are a few ways to work it out:

- Take a step back when you feel you're about to explode. Instead of ripping your spouse's head off, find a way to focus on what you love about him. Think of great times you've spent together and the qualities you hope your new child will inherit from him, and share this information with him.
- Try to get away from all the "baby stuff": the OB appointments, the registry at Babies "Я" Us, the nursery decorating. Allow yourselves to have some quality time alone. A lot of couples steal away for a last-chance vacation—otherwise known as a "babymoon"—before the baby is born (see chapter 9). You can also go out on a date night or cuddle on the couch and watch Netflix. The important thing is to take the time to reconnect and relax.
- Acknowledge that this is a stressful time in your lives—but you have each other to get through it, together. Practice patience and understanding (it will come in handy when you're parents) and put yourself in your partner's shoes.
- Don't sweat the small stuff. This was a big lesson for me, the eternal control freak. My fuse was so short, the tiniest thing that Cory did "wrong" or failed to do could set me off on a tirade. I'd yell—then I'd feel terrible. Was it really so earth-shattering that we were five minutes late to a party? Or that he left the toilet seat up again (grrrrr!). In the grand scheme of things, you as a couple is what

matters. You're a team—you'll both be up at the crack of dawn changing diapers and feeding the baby. You have each other's back, and that's what you should focus on.

"Honey, Can You Bring Me ... ?"

Earlier I mentioned that the one carrying the bambino seems to get her way. That doesn't mean that your man should feel like whatever you say goes. My mama always told me, "You get more flies with honey." Totally true. Men do not like to be told what to do. Your husband will feel used and abused, not willing to be your happy helper. A few clever techniques will make him want to cater to your every whim.

- **GUYS LOVE A CHALLENGE.** It makes them feel all smart and macho! When you're too exhausted or large to set up the nursery, try, "Sweetie, I just can't figure out how to put the crib together. It's so complicated!" Nothing motivates a man more than the old damsel-in-distress routine—plus he'll want to show how simple it is . . . for *him*. Not only will he put the crib together, he'll do it with lightning speed to prove his mental prowess. Sit back, put your feet up, and watch him drill and hammer to his heart's content.
- **ACTIONS SPEAK LOUDER THAN WORDS.** I wanted sex 24/7. But rather than throwing Cory down on the bed, I gave him

subtle hints. Grabbing his butt in public does not count. To get your point across in a truly subtle manner, when you're at dinner in a restaurant, stroke the inside of his wrist or run your toes up his pant leg. Rent a sexy, romantic movie, parade around the house in flimsy lingerie (yes, it comes in maternity sizes!), lick your lips, or simply hold his hand. Experts say touch stimulates the human bond. Touch him as much as possible!

- **GUILT HIM INTO IT.** An age-old technique perfected by our parents! Now's the time to turn it on your unsuspecting spouse. Say he wants to sit home on a Sunday and watch the football game, and you want to go out shopping for baby stuff. Start with a dramatic sigh, then say, "Oh, I am so stressed out about getting all the things I need for *our* baby before he comes . . ." Moan and groan, shake your head, choke back a few tears. Pour it on, girl! Then toss in for emphasis, "I have so little time to prepare before I have to deliver *our* child." Trust me, he'll be pushing that shopping cart in no time.

- **SHOWER HIM WITH PRAISE.** Every time your hubby does something helpful, tell him what a great job he did: "Honey, the dishes sparkle! You rock!" It's like scratching your dog behind the ears when he heels at your command: "Good boy! Good boy!" He'll feel appreciated and heroic, and you'll get regular foot rubs and someone to pick up towels off the bathroom floor when you're too big to bend over.

- **TELL HIM.** By this I mean: Communicate. Your guy is not a mind reader. He won't know that you want/desperately need a pepperoni pizza at two a.m. unless you verbalize. Case in point: I was feeling anxious—*very* anxious, a few days before my C-section. Cory was cool as a cucumber. I wanted him to calm my nerves, assure me everything would be okay. I needed comfort and affection. What I needed was a hug! Instead, I was biting my nails in silence, trying to be strong. Finally, I spoke up: "It'll be okay, right?" I asked. Cory put his arms around me (no easy task, considering I was so rotund!). "It's gonna be fine," he said. And I believed him and heaved a huge sigh of relief. I only wished I had asked him sooner—I would have felt a lot better!

- **POINT OUT THE PERKS.** Never underestimate the enticement of a reward. If you want something done, show your man what he will get out of it. For example, you need to clean out the garage to make room for the three baby strollers you bought. Explain that by clearing the space, he'll have more room to store his golf clubs, his old collection of 45s, a new sports car . . .

- **TIMING IS EVERYTHING.** Men have mood swings just like women! Some wake up cranky; some melt down midday; others are exhausted and unyielding at night. You want to bring up the topic of converting his man cave into a playroom when he's least irritable. My advice is to wait until the weekend when he's relaxing or when he's had a particularly great day at the office. Make sure he's eaten (preferably his fave meal). Take his emotional temperature before you spring anything on him.

His Turn: How to Make Your Pregnant Wife Happy

Cory was a saint when I was pregnant: he made me breakfast, lunch, and dinner when I was on bed rest my last month. He also did the grocery shopping and tidied up the house, washed the dishes, took the trash out, picked up and dropped off my mail. And when I couldn't tie my shoes or shave my legs, he did that as well. He liked to joke that he was my "weed whacker." So romantic.

For all your well-meaning men out there, he offers the following words of wisdom:

DON'T...

- Tell her she looks fat (yeah, she knows that already).
- Tell her she looks tired (yeah, she knows that, too).
- Compare her with other pregnant women. As in: "How come Joe's wife never pukes and always looks great?" She's having *your* baby, and you gotta deal with it.
- Tell her you know how she's feeling. 'Cause you don't. Not even a little. And this just pisses her off.
- Expect her to be rational. She is not the woman you married; she has been temporarily chemically altered. She may scream, cry, or burst into hysterical laughter at any given moment. Get used to it.
- Act nervous or anxious. A pregnant woman needs her man to be a calm, steady rock—not a bundle of nerves. So if you have to, fake it.

DO . . .

- Rub her feet, her back, anything that aches. Instant brownie points, brother.

- Clean up around the house without being asked. You think she can actually bend over to pick up that towel you dropped?

- Go to OB appointments. Unless she asks you not to. Always assume she will need a hand to hold, and frankly, since it's not you in the stirrups, it's the least you can do!

- Be thoughtful. Serve her breakfast in bed, draw her a bubble bath, bring home flowers. Or best yet, say *I love you*. Amazing what those three little words can do.

- Buy her stuff. I'm not just talking diapers or a breast pump, I'm talking a goodie now and then. A cupcake, flowers, and even a "push present" (a gift for pushing out that baby!) as a generous show of love and appreciation for all she's been going through.

- Make sure she has food and water at all times. Your spouse will get very, very cranky if she's hungry or thirsty. Fair warning.

- Nod and say, "Yes, dear," at all times. It will save you both a lot of pain if you simply agree with everything she says (even if you don't).

Ask the OB

Is it true that your hubby can feel sympathy pains and nausea and may gain weight when you're preggers?

It's true! Guys can have pregnancy symptoms, too. There's even a medical term for it. Couvade syndrome is a phenomenon where an otherwise healthy expectant father experiences physical symptoms and pains associated with his wife's pregnancy—the most common of which include weight gain, nausea, heartburn, appetite changes, disruption in sleep patterns, backaches, itchy skin, and in extreme cases labor pains or postpartum depression. Some studies estimate that as many as 80 percent of fathers-to-be develop at least one pregnancy-like symptom.

For most men affected, the symptoms appear toward the latter half of the pregnancy, although they have been known to occur as early as the end of the first trimester. The syndrome is largely believed to be psychosomatic, but the symptoms are very real for the men who are experiencing them. So take it as a compliment—he's being sympathetic to your suffering! It's sweet—as long as he doesn't expect you to start rubbing his achy feet.

I Get By with a Little Help from My Friends

I don't know what I would have done without my *Game* pals to get me through this pregnancy.

The Game party animal Hosea is a hoot. He tells it to me like it is, and he loves to bust my chops: "You'd think you're the only woman who's ever been pregnant before," he chided me. "I got news for you . . . you're not the first and you won't be the last—so quit the complaining!"

"Am I fat?" I asked him. I asked everyone—but I knew he would give it to me straight.

"You didn't give me the memo today: should I lie to you or not?" He laughed. "Of course you're fat! You're pregnant!"

"I'm scared I'm going back to work on the show six weeks after I give birth, and I'm going to be heavy."

"You are. You're not gonna lose that weight that quick—get that through your head. No one will notice: we'll camouflage your big ol' butt."

He brought over lunch another day, but wouldn't let me have any. "You are especially large and ridiculously unproportioned," he teased. But he did get me a cupcake!

By the end of our lunch, I was laughing my head off and feeling so much better. Hosea's like my girlfriend. Cory sometimes gets jealous: "You're on the phone with him for forty minutes!" But I just can't help it—we always love to gab and gossip, and I know he has my back (as long as it doesn't require babysitting duty).

Oh, Baby!

Another one of my great friends from *The Game*, Wendy, gasped when she saw me in my third trimester. "You look like you're in a fat suit! Where's Tia?"

I started to laugh so hard I went into contractions. "It's just Braxton-Hicks," I told her.

"Toni Braxton? You got Toni Braxton in there?"

"No, Braxton-Hicks are false labor pains!"

I was cracking up. But I also wanted to get serious with my friend: "I don't want a cesarean," I told her. "It adds two extra weeks to the recovery, and I won't be able to work out."

"You're going to be fine. Everything happens for a reason. Consider it a blessing," she told me. And for the first time in a long time, I felt a little better about my situation. Thanks, Wend!

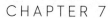

CHAPTER 7

Way Too Much Information

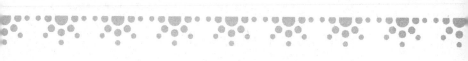

Today my sis and I settled on my couch with a bowl of popcorn for a little entertainment. We were going to watch Ricki Lake's documentary, The Business of Being Born. So many women were telling me about this film, I had to see it. Ricki says her birth was "an indescribable high."

"I guess if I'm considering doing this at home, I should see what I'm in for," I told Tamera. So we pressed Play, and there was Ricki. And I mean ALL of Ricki. OMG!

"Oh, no!" Tamera shrieked, covering her eyes. "Is that her . . ."

"Yes!" I couldn't stop staring in disbelief. Why did I want to see this? Ricki was in a bathtub, in her apartment, and it did not look like she was having fun. The pushing, the pain, the blood! We screamed! It was worse than Friday the 13th!

"Okay, I just made up my mind," I gasped, "I am having this kid in a hospital."

Tamera nodded. "And I just made up my mind to use birth control!"

I still figured I should get Cory's opinion on this important part of my birth plan. He watched a few seconds of the video and was scared out of his wits, worse than Tamera or I had been.

"You cannot be considering this!" he exclaimed. "This is too much to go through."

I was so touched that my honey didn't want me to suffer. Then he added, "Not for you . . . for me!"

The Write Stuff . . . or Is It?

When I found out I was pregnant (okay, maybe while I was trying to conceive—wishful thinking!), I read every book I could get my hands on and diligently surfed the Web, trying to understand what was in store for me. There was a ton of conflicting info out there. I read more than twenty pregnancy books, each with its own angle. (One of my favorites was *Preggatinis: Mixol-*

ogy for the Mom-to-Be.) But what particularly bugged me was that there was rarely anyone who looked like me in these books. Hello? African-American women get pregnant, too!

I turned to my computer for a more varied set of views, and found that everyone and their mother had something to say. Here's what I learned. Blogs and online message boards are filled with personal opinions based on individual experience. I appreciate it when moms share their knowledge, but I also realize that every pregnancy is different. Case in point: One chick insisted the best way to bring on labor was to park her ten-months-pregnant butt on a playground swing and pump her legs in the air. Her water broke within seconds. Hope there were no kids around!

Ask the OB

I've read every book and can't seem to get a straight answer on this one. Can I drink tea, coffee, or alcohol when I'm pregnant?

One cup of a caffeinated beverage (coffee or tea) per day has no known harmful effects on the baby. More than that isn't good for the fetus. And by one cup, I don't mean the triple-large coffee with an extra shot of espresso. It's important to be aware that decaf coffee isn't "caffeine-free." It has about 3 percent of the caffeine in a cup of regular coffee, about as much as in one or two cups of regular tea. Also, green tea can contain as much caffeine as a small espresso; just because the package says something is "herbal" doesn't mean the contents are caffeine-free. Read your labels carefully and don't be afraid to ask questions.

When it comes to alcohol, just stay away from it. Alcohol consumption during pregnancy can lead to a wide range of mental and physical birth defects. Though most women know that heavy drinking is bad, most don't realize that moderate or even light drinking can be harmful to a fetus. In fact, there is no level of alcohol that has been proven safe. Stick to the sparkling apple cider; the risk just isn't worth it.

Go ahead and read if it makes you feel smarter, better prepared, or less alone in this process. But don't let it psych you out. The more I watched and read during my pregnancy, the more I became aware that too much knowledge can be a bad thing. It can cause you sleepless nights of worry; it can confuse you; it can make you want to throw your laptop out the window (I came pretty close). This isn't to say you should bury your head in the sand. Just don't fill your head with conflicting facts and figures and nightmare scenarios.

Learn to filter. The book that suggested I burn incense and perform a Kundalini chant if the labor pains got too intense? Recycling bin. The article about increased sensation during sex in the last trimester? That was a keeper. I suggest you make yourself an informed mama-to-be, but beware the subjects that push your buttons. For me, it was anything about pain: cramping, constipation, cutting you open during a C-section. Just writing about this makes me feel a little woozy! So I would cheerfully skip those chapters in any book, or change the channel if someone on *The Doctors* was talking about episiotomies. I just did not want to think about being in agony. All I wanted to hear from friends, family, and my OB was that it would be a walk in the park—and if it wasn't, then I would be drugged enough not to know what hit me. Other mamas might want to know the gory details. I preferred to be blissfully ignorant.

One of my girlfriends also warned me about watching baby shows on TV: "Do not allow yourself to watch even one minute of *Baby Story*, *Bringing Home Baby*, or *One Born Every Minute*," she said. "It will give you nightmares." Aw, come on—how could a show starring an adorable little newborn make me anxious?

I should have known better. I am a TV actress and I know television will always be television. Drama, conflict, and gore equal higher ratings. One day I was flipping channels when I happened upon a baby-show marathon. I made myself a bowl of popcorn and settled in for a fun triple feature. I was horrified! Every single episode presented the scary side of pregnancy—all the stuff that could and did go wrong. A lady delivered in the back of a taxi! A woman developed a massive infection after delivery! A preemie was born weighing three pounds! After four straight hours of watching, I was a wreck. Some actually showed the C-section! There were surgeons! There were scalpels! There were stomach staples! I never knew childbirth involved office supplies!

How to Educate Yourself About Pregnancy (Without Losing Your Marbles)

I am normally an anxious person. By this I mean I am more likely to envision the worst-case scenario—and be convinced it's going to happen to me. Usually, I'm not too far off (we refer to it as Tia's Law). Most of the time I can laugh it off when something goes wrong, but when I became pregnant, my daily angst was amplified and much harder to handle. Every kick, cramp, or question mark became a crisis: "I am an insane pregnant woman! Give me an ultrasound now!"

I wanted to know what was going to happen, and it gave me some comfort initially to be able to take the reins by studying up. I learned the physiology of pregnancy and charted my baby's development every week. I felt organized and empowered. But as the pregnancy progressed and it became more real to me (there is actually a baby growing in my stomach!), less was more. Since there was no avoiding what I was in for, I didn't want to know about it. I didn't want to mull over every horrible complication that could arise. Too much information was making me nuts. When I started spouting pregnancy stats ("Forty-eight percent of all women experience morning sickness!"), I knew it was time to stop. Was this information useful to me? Did it give me relief or comfort or make me stop vomiting (fat chance!). I decided I would rather be on a need-to-know basis with my pregnancy. The stuff that could keep me and my baby healthy was what I would take in. Details on the surgical instruments used during delivery, I would skip. Some ladies will disagree with me on this; they want to know every detail. That's fine if you can stomach it. I was barely keeping down my breakfast—the last thing I needed was to learn the length of the amnio needle. If I could have gone through the majority of my OB appointments blindfolded, I probably would have been better off!

Pregnancy is an exercise in faith, girlfriend. It's out of your hands. You can't 100 percent control it or predict how it will go—nor can your doctor. You are totally trusting the universe to be kind and spare you as much pain and suffering as possible. No matter how prepared you think you are, no matter how careful and diligent, stuff happens. And amazingly, it can all change in a split second. When I reached my last trimester, my OB informed me that the baby was breech, and there was little we could do to change this. I racked my brain: Had I done something to make the baby face the wrong way, feet first?

"No, Tia," Dr. Kumetz reassured me. "It's nothing you did. He's just in this position, and he may move. Or he may not."

There it was: No control. I couldn't fix the problem, even if I read every article about how to turn a breech baby and tried everything they suggested (even pointing a flashlight up my you-know-what!). My relatively normal, healthy pregnancy had turned into a possible emergency situation. We scheduled a C-section. All that info I had taken in during my delivery classes was for nothing? I had memorized all the stages of labor, and now I would not be experiencing it. That irritated me, but I didn't beat myself up over it. I felt like I had done my very best to ensure my baby would come into this world healthy. I was always a girl who did her homework. It was a change of plans, but it would be okay. And the last thing I wanted to read about now was C-section births! Instead, I read children's books to my baby. According to Dr. Oz, fetuses hear voices filtered through tissue, bones, and fluid. And by week 24, they recognize—and are calmed by—their mothers' voices. Now, that was some info I could use!

Ask the OB

Will listening to music or reading to my baby make him smarter when he's born?

It's a great question, and an interesting theory, but the answer is no one knows for sure. There are medical studies that indicate a baby can hear and react to sound by moving, but no one really understands what those movements mean. There haven't been any studies done on the effects of sound stimulation of fetuses before birth and their intelligence, creativity, or neurologic development later in life. But if it makes you feel closer and more bonded with your baby, it can't hurt!

The Alien on My Sonogram

Sonograms in 3-D are promoted as a "picture perfect" way to see your new baby in utero—suitable for framing! As an actress, I love a good photo op, so I was totally game. Yes, it cost about double what a regular, 2-D sonogram cost—but you got two free four-by-sixes to share with friends and family. You could even buy a DVD of the images with a lullaby soundtrack!

Three-dimensional ultrasound sounded very cool: instead of sending the sound waves straight down and reflected back, they are sent at different angles. The returning echoes are processed by a high-tech computer program that reconstructs a 3-D image of the fetus, so you can see height, width, and depth—kind of like watching a 3-D movie. The baby's image "pops out" more, and it's supposed to give you a truer image of what your child will look like.

I was sold. Cory had an important audition, and I figured I'd fill him in and bring the beautiful pics home to frame. I was shocked when the doctor handed me my souvenir snapshot. I had expected an adorable baby boy. But my picture was of some strange, straggly creature from another planet. It wasn't cute or cuddly; it was kind of scary.

"Is this normal?" I asked. "I mean, is he supposed to look like this?"

The doctor assured me everything was developing the way it should at the twenty-week mark.

I brought the pictures home (hiding a few that were particularly horrific) and showed them to Cory. He totally freaked. I was glad I hadn't brought him with me; I think he might have passed out on the floor of the doctor's office.

"Oh my God!" he said, staring at the image of our baby. "What is wrong with him? He looks like an alien! What are all those weird bumps? Where are his ears? What's that weird bulge on his head? He looks deformed!"

"No, he's fine," I assured him. "It's supposed to look like that."

"Like E.T.?" Cory gasped. "My son looks like E.T.?"

Yeah, I could kind of see the resemblance: big head, scrawny body, long fingers. My poor husband had been looking forward to a handsome first photo of his son to carry in his wallet. Instead, he got something more along the lines of *The X-Files*. In retrospect, I wish someone had warned us that the 3-D sono wasn't something we needed to see. Instead of reassuring us, it made us worry for twenty more weeks that our son would look more like a Martian than like his mom or dad. Technology can be a good thing, but it can also give you results you don't expect. I am happy to report that Cree was perfectly healthy and beautiful when he was born—even if his first photo session wasn't a Kodak moment.

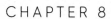

CHAPTER 8

Hot Mama

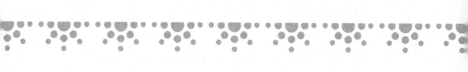

I'm not ready to start wearing one of those "with bump, not plump!" pregnancy tees, but my body sure is. Nothing's fitting, but the thought of a maternity muumuu is keeping me from going shopping. I'm going to need to figure something out—quick. I feel like I'm exploding out of every outfit. I had no idea that the rest of your body grows along with your belly (could my butt be pregnant, too?). I look at my sis—who is shaping up for her wedding and is looking so slim and sexy—and I could just bawl. We used to look like twins. Now I look like Tamera on helium . . .

*I*f I had to sum up my fashion philosophy pre-pregnancy, I could do it in one word: sexy. Everything I wore was about showing off my curves. I loved the shape I was in, thanks to my new diet and exercise, and frankly, my feeling is that you're not young forever. If you got it, honey, flaunt it—before gravity sets in. So, yes, I went for very va-va-voom looks: short, figure-hugging, cleavage-baring. I barely had a pair of heels less than four inches high, and I liked it that way. My wardrobe choices made me feel beautiful, strong, and feminine. My style was a bit bold and adventurous, and I swore that even when I was big as a house, I would not compromise that.

So I had a heart-to-heart with my stylist of seven years, Alexis Beck: "I wanna be a hot mama," I pleaded with her. "Help me!"

It was easy in the beginning. When I was barely showing, clothes that were one or two sizes bigger could easily camouflage my tiny baby bump. My cup size was growing, but I wasn't complaining about that (and neither was Cory!). I just needed to make sure I had the right support and used a bit of double-sided tape now and then to keep the girls in their place. In the second trimester, things got much tougher. Zippers wouldn't zip, buttons popped open, and I couldn't squeeze my rear end into anything in my closet. I was really depressed.

Is It Okay to Wear Tight Clothes While I'm Pregnant— Could It Hurt the Baby?

Pregnancy can sometimes be hard on your body image, and some women have difficulty accepting that their bodies are changing, especially when they are getting bigger. There is no evidence that wearing tight clothes will hurt the baby. The baby itself is well protected by many layers of muscle, the uterus, and amniotic fluid, but tight-fitting clothing, especially at the waist, can cause other discomforts during pregnancy. Heartburn, or acid reflux, is common during pregnancy, because of slower transit of food through the digestive tract due to the increase in progesterone. As the uterus grows and pushes the stomach and intestines up under the diaphragm, the risk of food's flowing upward increases. Pressure from tight clothing can exacerbate this effect, worsening heartburn.

I called Alexis for help. If I tried to go with even larger sizes that stretched over my belly, the proportions were all wrong. I showed her a dress that fit across my hips but had shoulders so big and wide that I looked like I was wearing a clown suit.

"You know what this means," she told me. "It's time for maternity clothes."

Ugh. The very words conjured up images of frumpy, dumpy, itchy, shapeless polyester dresses that tied in the back.

"I don't want to lose myself because I'm pregnant," I insisted. "I don't want to look matronly."

Alexis assured me that wouldn't happen. She warned me that if I continued buying huge, oversize clothes, people would think I was bingeing, not expecting. Well, that convinced me! We reached out to several designers and maternity stores, searching for styles that were "Tia-riffic." I was actually pleasantly surprised at what was out there. Isabella Oliver started as a maternity designer but also has a sportswear collection, and she was a godsend! Comfortable and chic. I loved her wraparound tops, ruched dresses, and long tunics (isabellaoliver.com/maternity-clothes). We also discovered that there were several designers who were making maternity clothing for A Pea in the Pod (apeainthepod.com), such as 7 For All Mankind denim, True Religion denim, and Joie. The clothes were fashion-forward and flattering, and übermom Heidi Klum designs a budget-friendly line of basics for A Pea in the Pod called Lavish (almost all the pieces are under $100).

I also loved Rachel Pally jersey dresses (rachelpally.com); they're perfect for before, during, and after pregnancy and come in bright colors and patterns that skim the body. It's no wonder that stars like Sarah Jessica Parker and Angelina Jolie love them. An empire waist worked well for me; it pushed up and covered my boobs and showed off my bump without making me look enormous. I stocked up on Rachel Pally strapless maxi dresses and lived in them those last, brutal weeks, when I felt so uncomfortable. At that point, style took a backseat to comfort: I just wanted to walk around naked all the time. Anything that was binding, pinching, or remotely tight . . . I couldn't bear to wear it. So these long, flowy gowns were just about the only thing I wanted to put on. Alexis helped me doll them up with accessories, and I looked fairly chic (if I do say so myself) in my inflated state.

The Agony of "De Feet"

Unfortunately, one of my style staples went out the window midway during my pregnancy: heels. All the gorgeous stilettos I had loved pre-mommyhood now hurt like hell. I tried to squeeze my swollen toes into them, but walking even a few steps made my back hurt. So Alexis let me in on a fashion secret: Flats can be sexy. Who knew there were so many glitzy, cute, fun ones out there? I wanted to buy them all—in every color! And in several sizes (my feet swelled daily, so I never knew what size I would be when I woke up). Besides being beautiful, they felt so good! I never dreamed I'd be wearing flat gladiator sandals with a long evening gown to my sister's wedding, but they looked hot! Even now that I *can* be back in heels, I've been opting to stay closer to the ground. I feel like a new woman, and you should see my shoe collection these days. Not just colors and patterns, but every heel height imaginable! If you're a girl who just can't give up your heels, try wedges: they'll give you extra inches but are much sturdier.

Mama Wardrobe Must-Haves

Style is very personal—and that goes for maternity fashion as well. I can tell you only what worked for me, because every body is different. My best advice is to try stuff on. Those pregnancy pillows they have in dressing rooms really do help you gauge how you'll look weeks down the road. After a few panicky moments, I tried not to obsess about how big my belly was getting. Alexis told me, "A baby is flattering on everyone." It's true: in the right outfit, I did feel powerful and regal sporting my bump.

Every woman stresses over how she looks when she's pregnant. You've never seen yourself this way, and it feels freaky—especially when you have no control over it. But rather than panic, remember that this is all temporary. You won't always look like a beach ball. Your body, with a little work, will go back to the way it was before. Part of the stress stems from everything changing all at once: your body, your health, your life. It's a lot to take in. Thank God for my sis, who constantly reminded me that no matter what I looked like on the outside, I was still the same person on the inside. And major kudos to my hubby for telling me how much he loved my big booty!

On a more positive note, being pregnant gives you a whole new reason to shop—as if I needed more reasons! Alexis helped me assemble a go-to wardrobe of pregnancy basics that I could dress up, dress down, or just crawl into to feel comfy. If you invest in these pieces, you'll be set for the next nine months . . . and then some.

- **A CLASSIC BLAZER.** Nothing looks more professional or polished. As your belly grows, you can simply wear it open and no one will be the wiser. I paired mine with everything from a dress to jeans, and it looked great. You can opt for a dark color, since it will go with anything, or pick a nice neutral, like white or beige, if it's summer or you live somewhere warm like L.A.

- **A LONG JERSEY DRESS.** As I said, Rachel Pally's worked great for me. You want to find one with a smooth, stretchy fabric that has a lot of give. I know it's tempting to buy everything in black (it hides all evils), but I think a shot of color can do wonders for your mood. Alexis and I tried to stay away from any dresses that were dark. I love bright shades like orange, red, and royal blue. Choose a neckline that flatters you—for me, it was either a V-neck, a wrap, or strapless with an empire cut. If your boobs are big, you want to go for an open neck—nothing too buttoned-up or blouson. It will only emphasize what you've got going on upstairs, and not in a good way! Choose the sleeves (or no sleeves) based on the season and your climate. When the rest of my bod was swollen beyond recognition, my arms and shoulders still looked toned. So I almost always wore sleeveless or strapless dresses to flaunt them.

- **A WRAP SWEATER.** When it was chilly at night or on an air-conditioned flight, I loved to pull one of these on. You can tie it as tight or as loose as you like, and it makes you look like you actually have a waist when you don't!

- **A CARDIGAN OR SHRUG.** A great topper, and layering helps when you're not sure whether you're going to feel hot one minute and cold the next. I got a bunch in different colors, then wore them over dresses, tanks, and tees. An easy way to inject a little color and excitement into your outfit while balancing out your heavier bottom half. A neutral is the most versatile (white, black, navy, beige), but I think a bright color over a simple black sheath is so chic. I'd suggest buying one that's lightweight (cotton or jersey), and one that's toastier (cashmere or wool).

- **A BEAUTIFUL SHAWL.** A gorgeous wrap takes any outfit to the next level. I grew to love mine like a favorite blanket. You can choose a simple, inexpensive pashmina or two in bright hues. I found some in funky boho patterns and florals that were really eye-catching. I also appreciated how this lovely, long piece of fabric covered me up when I was feeling huge.

- **TRAPEZE TANKS.** There were days when I couldn't stand anything that clung. Alexis found me some easy, breezy A-line tanks that I could wear with anything. I was always happy to show off my arms, so these became one of my favorite maternity staples. I love them now, even after I've delivered, because they're so comfy and cool.

- **A GREAT PAIR OF JEANS.** You may pay a bit more for a designer maternity pair, but it's so worth it. Your stomach won't go down immediately after you deliver (it's been months and I'm still waiting!), so you can continue wearing them. Most are made with a stretchy waist and belly band but look normal and flattering in the butt and legs. I found several 7 For All Mankind jeans at Pea in the Pod that were so comfy and made me feel "normal"—so I bought them in denim, white, and black. Boot-cut and a dark wash are the most flattering.

- **AN LMBD.** A little maternity black dress. I love the site moreofmematernity.com because they have such a huge assortment, everything from minis to maxis and every length in between. The Greek goddess one-shouldered style is very chic and sophisticated, as is the asymmetrical ruffled neckline. Pretty, comfy, and appropriate for any occasion.

The Finishing Touch

No matter what you're wearing, there are going to be days when you just feel like you wish you could wear a tent. And that, my friend, is what accessories are for!

- *Gold bangle bracelets.* I am comfortable wearing big, bold jewelry, so Alexis suggested I stock up on some statement pieces. I felt like I could pull on a stack and instantly add oomph to my outfit. Another plus: These are timeless and you will wear them well after your pregnancy. Plus Cree now loves the jingle-jangle sound they make!
- *Large hoop earrings.* I was obsessed with earrings, especially shoulder dusters, since they drew the eye up and away from my hips! Big hoops are a good bet, since you

can wear them casual or dressy. LL Cool J's wife, Simone I. Smith, makes some of my faves: delicate yet dramatic in both silver and gold (simoneismith.com).

- *A fabulous bag.* I liked to go bigger with my hobo purse when I was pregnant, because (a) I had a ton more to carry around with me, like snacks, water, and Burt's Bees Mama Bee Belly Balm, and (b) the bigger the bag, the smaller I looked! Just keep in mind that chain link and stud details—no matter how chic—will be heavy to begin with. As you get larger, your back will hurt and you're not going to want to be lugging around fifty pounds of hardware on your shoulder.

- *Ballet flats.* These are so ladylike and comfy at the same time, and you can wear them with a skirt or pants. Again, here's your chance to jazz up your outfit. Buy shoes in bright colors or adorned with buckles or accents. I carried a pair of Tory Burch Reva flats in my purse all the time—in case of emergencies! Remember that your feet will swell, so don't buy them too small, or they'll rub. I also really loved flat sandals and thongs, mainly because it felt better for me to let my poor, swollen toes breathe! Again, it's all about the details: you can find lots of inexpensive, strappy pairs with rhinestones, beads, even fringe. I definitely used my shoes to transform something as basic as a tank and skirt into a stylish ensemble. And the fancier your footwear, the more people will be looking at your feet and not your basketball of a belly!

What to Wear Under There

I could deal with my cup size growing, but when I realized my favorite pair of underwear (you know you've got 'em) was pinching and giving me a wedgie, it was time to consult the experts. For advice, I turned to the ladies of 2 Chix (2chix.com), a maternity boutique in Santa Monica with a great reputation for hot mama wear. They taught me that you have to "keep your lady parts happy" when you're preggers. But that does not mean granny panties (perish the thought!). Opt for comfortable *and* sexy!

- Try a low-rise boy short in either cotton or lacy styles— they'll be roomier in the hips, thighs, and waist and won't ride up. Buy one size up from your normal size for added comfort.
- For your top half, skip the pricey maternity bras and go wireless instead. Many of the major lingerie companies produce wireless bras that are both forgiving to your growing twins and gentle on the mammary glands (which is important if you're planning to breast-feed). Lightweight nylon/spandex seamless stretch bras are also light, comfy, and practical and can be found at many department stores and boutiques.
- If you're already well endowed and now bordering on OMG, then a traditional maternity bra may supply the best support. Just be sure to get properly fitted.

- Maternity Spanx. They don't call them Power Mama Shapers for nothin'. They also make full-length and foot-less pantyhose. They suck you in. Nuff said.

Pamper Yourself

Taking the time to make sure you look great on the outside does a wealth of good for your mental and emotional health. Manis, pedis, facials, blow-outs, massages. Do it! And if you can't or don't feel like going to a salon, invite your girlfriends over and take turns treating one another. You deserve it. All of it! The nicest thing my sissy ever did for me was bring a manicurist into my home when I was on bed rest to give me a mani–pedi. She painted my toes baby blue (for boy!) and I felt refreshed, re-vived, and renewed.

It was seriously a month and a half *after* I delivered before I had time/patience to get another mani–pedi. And if it weren't for the stylists on *The Game*, I'm pretty sure my hair would eternally be in a head scarf. Who has time to pamper yourself when you're changing a newborn's diapers every hour? So I am not kidding when I tell you to treat yourself to a spa day before you have the baby. Facial, massage, haircut, the works. It's good for both body and soul. Not only will you feel better, but you'll look less like crap in the hospital when people visit you. Eventu-ally, you'll be able to get your roots touched up and your eye-brows waxed, but don't count on it for at least a few weeks while baby gets settled in. Do all your beauty biz before the Big Day. You'll thank me later.

If you don't want to spend a fortune on a day spa, it's fine to just spoil yourself at home. I would light candles in my bathroom, sink into a scented bubble bath, and just Zen out whenever I felt the stress mounting. Ahhhh . . .

Ask the OB

I read in a pregnancy book that coloring your hair is dangerous for the baby. Am I supposed to go for nine months with a dull do?

OTIS (The Organization of Teratology Information Specialists), which provides information on potential reproductive risk, says that animal studies are reassuring and there are no reports of hair dye causing changes in human pregnancy. In addition, only a minimal amount of the chemicals in hair dye is actually absorbed into your system. So the limited evidence available suggests that it's probably safe to dye your hair during pregnancy. That being said, since the evidence is limited, I recommend waiting to dye your hair until your second trimester (14 weeks), when you are outside the window in which the fetus is the most vulnerable. Also, rather than all-over hair color, consider a process like highlighting, in which the chemicals have little or no contact with your scalp, and be sure to sit in a well-ventilated space to minimize breathing in the chemicals.

CHAPTER 9

Booty Call

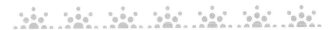

Suddenly, there's a threesome in my bed. I heard that guys do get a little freaked out, but the ironic thing is that I am horny all the time. It's some cruel trick of nature—these hormones are like Viagra on speed.

You'd think that with all the puking and belching I'd just want to be left alone, but the truth is, if Cory just looks at me I want to jump his bones!

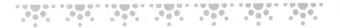

So last night, I had this wild, wicked dream about making love to my man. It was hot; it was dirty. I think there might have been a hot tub and massage oil involved. I woke up panting, sweating, biting my pillow. It was incredibly vivid, and for a split second, I thought it was real. Then I looked over to find Cory fast asleep next to me in the bed. I guess the part about the Reddi-wip was also a dream? It's crazy how much I think about sex. I don't even have to be awake for my brain to start fantasizing.

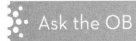

Ask the OB

Why do I have weird sex dreams when I'm pregnant?

Everyone dreams every night, whether they remember it the next day or not. There are several factors that work together during pregnancy that may increase dream recall and frequency. Libido, or sex drive—often the very cause of pregnancy—can undergo very dramatic swings during the nine months of gestation. Hormonal changes trigger extra blood flow to the breasts and genitals, which can increase sensitivity, sexual arousal, and the desire for sex. Dreams are also more readily recalled just upon waking, and since pregnancy can lead to waking up more frequently at night, there is a higher likelihood you will remember what the dream was about. And then there are the many emotions you are feeling in regard to the pregnancy. Since it is more difficult to be intimate in the last few months of pregnancy because of the expanding tummy, one theory is that the sex dreams might be an emotional compensation.

Once my bump started showing, when I talked about getting down and dirty, Cory was turned on but also very nervous. "Tia, take it down a notch," he'd say, as I purred like a kitten in his ear. "We're going to hurt the baby!" He actually worried he'd poke him with his you-know-what!

Experts will tell you that a woman's libido tends to go into overdrive as she hits the second trimester: that's because of increased blood flow to your sexual organs and breasts. Translation: I was a total horndog. The first time we had sex while I was pregnant, my hubby was a little skittish: "I feel like the baby is watching!" he whispered. I needed Cory to meet me at least halfway! It took a couples counseling visit to Dr. Kumetz to put his mind at ease. She told us it was absolutely, positively okay to get down and dirty. It wouldn't cause a miscarriage. It wouldn't poke the baby in the eye. The developing fetus is protected by the amniotic fluid in your uterus, as well as the mucus plug that blocks the cervix. At the most, orgasm could cause mild uterine contractions, generally temporary and harmless. We had the OB's blessing: hallelujah!

But as I grew larger, it became more logistically challenging to satisfy my needs. Poor Cory, it was like trying to make love to a blowfish! We tried to get creative. If missionary style no longer worked, there were a host of other positions that felt more comfy (see "Making Whoopee," below). It was also a lot of fun to experiment. I highly recommend that you get yourself a copy of one of the many editions of the *Kama Sutra*, *The Joy of Sex*, or some other book with diagrams. Check 'em off as you go along.

Making Whoopee . . . When You're the Size of a Beached Whale

Easy it isn't, but not only is sex good for your mood (it releases lots of natural endorphins), it helps you reconnect with your partner. Orgasm makes a happy mommy—which makes a happy baby! I never wanted sex as much as when I was pregnant! I had crazy fantasies and erotic dreams. Plus, pregnancy hormones make your ligaments lengthen, giving you more flexibility, and allowing you to put on your own Cirque du Soleil act in bed! I leave it to you to find your own groove, but "sexpert" moms-to-be (you know who you are!) recommend the following.

Mama on top. You can take the lead, moving whichever way feels good. Love it!

Side by side. You lie facing each other, and you can drape one leg over him. Not particularly effective in the third trimester (bump gets in the way), but a good choice up until then. And you can look into each other's eyes.

The spoon. He lies behind you and enters from behind. An intimate and gentle way to make love.

Take a seat. Straddle your partner's lap with your legs wrapped around him, as he sits on a sturdy, comfy chair. A good way to get in a quickie!

Oh, Baby!

Right behind you. Lean on a pillow while your partner enters you from behind. It's deep penetration, so take it slow—it can be intense!

Do You Think I'm Sexy?

It was the weekend of my sister's wedding in romantic wine country. My publicist, Jordyn, suggested I seize the moment. "Get away, just the two of you," she suggested. "Have a baby-moon!"

I did feel a little bad that with all the focus on the baby, I had been neglecting Cory. I was eight months pregnant; this might be our last chance to get away somewhere, just the two of us, for a long, long time.

I loved the idea! I dragged Tamera with me to buy sexy maternity lingerie that would make my man salivate. I found two naughty-but-nice outfits: a black-lace nightie and matching panties, and a colorful print silk kimono. In the dressing room, I imagined how Cory would undress me with his eyes. Then I turned around to take a look in the full-length mirror.

"Oh my God!" I screamed. "I look *huge!*" I was bawling while the saleslady tried to assure me that my butt didn't look as big as I thought it did. It was just the lighting in the dressing room! Yeah, right.

Bloated and blue, I packed my purchases for our trip, and some candles, and prayed that the lighting in our hotel room would be dim (a blackout wouldn't be bad, either). I broke the news to Cory in the car: "I thought maybe we could have a little fun this weekend, too. You know, a babymoon."

Cory looked puzzled: "Did you just make that up? I've never heard of that."

"No! It's real!" I insisted. "It's like a honeymoon . . . but with a very pregnant wife."

"Uh-huh," he replied. "Yeah, sure. I'm down for it."

But things didn't go exactly as planned. We got lost and wound up late to Tamera's rehearsal dinner (she was not too happy), and after a seven-hour drive in the car, my feet and legs swelled up and I was exhausted. All I wanted to do was sleep . . . not make whoopee.

Cory was understanding (and pretty exhausted himself). The babymoon never really happened the way I planned it (sensing a theme here?). But I did eventually get to unveil my lacy lingerie at a later time back home.

"Wow, baby, you look hot!" Cory exclaimed, whistling through his teeth, as I entered the bedroom.

"Really?" I replied. "This is hot to you?" Did I need to get my hubby's vision checked?

"Not just hot . . . sexy as hell!" He took me in his arms and pulled me down on the bed.

Go figure. While I was stressing about my girth, Cory actually got turned on by it. "There's more of you to love," he teased. Lesson learned: Men are blind when it comes to baby weight. Embrace your ballooning bod; feel sexy and confident. He won't be able to keep his hands off you . . . all of you.

Sex After Baby

Here's something they never tell you: Sex may not feel the same after you deliver. Some of the stuff you have down there has been stretched out, maybe even snipped or stitched. It's sore as hell. And thanks to decreasing estrogen, your vagina may suddenly feel as dry as the Sahara. Most OBs will say to hold off for at least four to six weeks to let yourself heal. But trust me . . . I was in no rush. While I was pregnant, all I could think about was sex. Now all I can think about is sleep! I'm a walking zombie most of the time, and that does little for the libido. I had no idea my sex drive could go from one hundred to zero in a matter of weeks!

That's why I strongly advocate having as much sex as possible while you're pregnant. After that adorable little munchkin comes along, it could be as long as a few months before you and your hubby get back to business—or you even want to. Just don't forget about the daddy. If you're not in the mood to have sex, then simply cuddle, hold hands, kiss. Take things slow—you'll be feeling the big O again before you know it! And I promise you, it does get better. Just wait till your little bundle of joy is sleeping through the night, and suddenly it's just you and your man in bed, in the dark. Even if it takes a while, it's like riding a bike, girlfriend—you never forget how to do it!

Exercising Your Equipment

My trainer, Jeanette, also taught me some great Kegel or pelvic-floor exercises that are good for keeping everything down there strong and tight (especially handy when you're ready to have sex again!). Kegels improve circulation to your vagina and rectum, so they also help speed healing after childbirth. Another plus: If you pee every time you laugh or sneeze, this will help strengthen the muscles so you don't leak!

At first I giggled when Jeanette instructed me on how to do them. Seriously? My va-jay-jay needs a workout? She told me I could do them anywhere, anytime. This cracked me up. But if you're doing it right, no one will be able to tell. I think it's a great thing to do when you're stuck in traffic... or waiting in the dentist's office... or watching the evening news... or brushing your teeth...

How to do a Kegel

1. Imagine yourself peeing—now try to stop the flow of urine midstream. Squeeze and lift the muscles. At first you may have trouble isolating these pelvic-floor muscles, but it gets easier with practice.

2. Start by holding each contraction for a few seconds before you release it. Relax a few seconds after each one. As your muscles get stronger, you'll be able to hold each Kegel for about 10 seconds. Do them in sets of 10 and try to work up to 3 or 4 sets about 3 times a day.

3. Check your form: You shouldn't be tightening your tummy, your buttocks, or your legs, or holding your breath. Only your pelvic-floor muscles should be moving.

Making Time to Make Love

Between work and taking care of Cree, I realize my hubby is getting the short end of the stick. There's only so much of me to go around! But here's the thing: You have to make sex a priority in your life. Your partner may already feel like a third wheel because you're so focused on the baby. He needs a little attention, too!

Even if you're both tired; even if you're both stressed; even if you have only a few minutes while the baby is taking a nap . . . seize the moment. I know a lot of couples actually schedule sex time every few days. I can't do this; I don't turn on like a lightbulb. I need a little romance, a little spontaneity. So there is a lot to be said for a quickie! Some couples don't even mind if the baby is in the room. (Personally, this puts a damper on the passion for Cory. He doesn't like an audience!) In our case, we've had to get creative with the where and when. I highly recommend it—it puts the excitement back into your sex life.

Here's where you might be able to find a few minutes:

- In the kitchen while you're waiting for the pasta water to boil

- During halftime break when watching Sunday football
- While you're doing the laundry (there's something very sexy about the spin cycle, don't you think?)
- When the grandparents are busy oohing and ahhing over the baby (they'll be busy, so you can get busy in the bedroom!)
- At the break of dawn before you get up to start the day
- When baby learns to sleep through the night. Make sure you two don't!

CHAPTER 10

Bugaboos, Boppies, and Bottles—Oh, My!

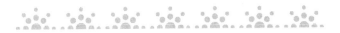

I cannot wait to shop for my baby! I already have a list: swing, stroller, bassinet, crib, bottles, blankets, clothes, bibs, diapers, car seat . . .

Hmm . . . we may need a bigger place . . . But, that said, raising a kid shouldn't cost a million dollars. Though I'm tempted to buy everything for my little bundle of joy, I know one little baby can't possibly need or use all this stuff!

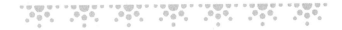

*T*amera threw me a huge baby shower at The London hotel in West Hollywood. I have to admit: I wasn't looking forward to my shower. I was pretty uncomfortable—entering the "get this baby out of me" stage, and completely stressed about all my friends seeing me so large at nine months. When I watch myself now on *Tia & Tamera*, I swear I don't recognize that swollen chick waddling around on camera! Where did my feet go? My chin?

The shower was mid-June and I was due late June; this was not a time when I wanted all the attention—nor did I particularly love being on camera. But because of Tamera's wedding and shooting our show, this was when we could fit in my baby shower.

Auntie-to-be Tamera, on the other hand, was very excited, and I tried not to burst her bubble.

"It will be so much fun—just think of all the presents!" she gushed. All I could think was, *Maybe I can hide my huge belly and booty behind the gifts?*

But once I was there, I relaxed. It was great to see all my friends, especially Jackée, who is like a second mom to me (she played my mom on *Sister, Sister*). And I did leave with tons of baby loot: everything from burp cloths to bottle warmers; infant designer jeans (who knew they made them that small!) to Whoozits (bizarre-looking Velcro creatures you strap to a stroller or crib).

After the shower, I surveyed everything I had received and bought for the baby. As I sat in my house, surrounded by mountains of infant paraphernalia, I wondered how much of this I would actually use or need. It seemed like a lot of stuff for one little person!

You won't really know what you'll need till you bring the baby home. And expect the unexpected—I've had friends buy the hospital-certified breast pump, only to find themselves rushing to the store for cases of formula when they found out the baby was allergic to everything but. This isn't meant to overwhelm you, but to explain that despite all the checklists from magazines and maternity stores—and I wound up checking them *all* off, which kind of defeated the purpose—ultimately it's you who will figure out what your baby's basic needs are.

There's definitely no harm in trying to prepare, but trust me, you'll be tempted to believe every ad for a new baby product, and all those nice registry helpers who tell you that you can't make do with just one stroller. I don't want to spoil your fun shopping for all those adorable, tiny baby goodies. I'm just saying if you don't want to buy everything, you don't have to. A newborn needs very little. You're stressed out enough about delivering—you don't need to max out your credit cards on top of that.

Having been through it, from the rush of the first trip to the baby store, to the seventh trip to return something, here—in my humble opinion—is what you really need and really don't.

ADD THESE TO YOUR REGISTRY

- **A DOZEN ONESIES.** The simple cotton ones are best, preferably with snaps or Velcro in the crotch for easy diaper changing. This is the baby equivalent of you wearing your fave T-shirt to bed. It's comfy and easy. You could probably survive on five to seven, but I hate to do laundry. I also found myself changing Cree's three to five times a day—my little man is the king of spit-up. And no matter how many adorable ensembles my sis or mom bought him, it's just easier for both of us if he wears a onesie.

- **THREE OR FOUR EASY SWADDLING BLANKETS.** Swaddling your child makes him feel like he's cozy in the womb. To be honest, doing it with a regular receiving blanket takes some origami skills. I am up to my eyeballs in blankies— big ones, small ones, ones with choo-choos and bunnies all over them. Frankly, the only one I need is the Summer Infant SwaddleMe (about $10.99 for the fleece one; $27.99 for a cotton three-pack on Amazon.com). It comes with a little "pocket" that you can tuck baby into, and Velcro to secure his arms so he's toasty warm. Makes it so much easier to swaddle him in the middle of the night in the dark. The foot part also drops down, so you can do a quickie change. And he looks like a cute little baby burrito in it!

- **A STUFFED ANIMAL THAT PLAYS SOOTHING SOUNDS.** Amid all the giant plush teddy bears, Clifford the Dogs, and hippos twice the size of Cree, I found an adorable Mama Bear who has a sound box that mimics what he heard in his mommy's tummy: gentle water whooshing and a comforting heartbeat ($24.99 at Toys "Я" Us). Works like a charm: I turn it on, and he's out cold. The elaborate mobile that Cory and I struggled to put together that plays a sleep-inducing lullaby? Cree lies there wide awake, staring at it!

- **A BABY MONITOR.** If you want a life, I strongly recommend you get one of these. You can go pee, make dinner, and work on your computer without hovering nervously over the crib, waiting for your baby to stir. Mine is supersensitive, so I can hear him breathing. You can carry it around with you or put a few receivers around the house. You can even spring for a high-tech one that comes with video as well as audio. Sometimes Cory and I just like to watch the monitor—better than pay-per-view! Most will run $50 to $100 (spring for the monitors that promise zero interference and work long-distance— otherwise you'll be listening to your neighbor's baby down the block); color monitors with night-vision cameras will run you double that.

- **A PACIFIER.** Otherwise known as a binky and Mom's best friend. I suggest you get yourself a bunch of these lovely little plastic nipples for your baby to suck on. You will always lose them; they will always pop out of his mouth and land somewhere filthy and germ-laden (you can boil them or sterilize them—but it grosses me out). Don't go crazy and buy too many, because you will soon find out that infants are binky-picky. You'll figure out the brand that makes him most happy—his least favorite he may actually spit across the room. Some are actually shaped like the real thing (and vaguely resemble something you'd find in a very different shop!). But the right one will soothe him during a meltdown and distract him when he's hungry (and you're frantically trying to warm the bottle). Make sure your pediatrician is cool with your baby's using one; there has been some concern over kids getting hooked on their pacifiers, and increased risk of middle-ear infections and dental problems. My pediatrician is fine with it, and I don't know about Cree, but I can't live without it!

- **A DIAPER PAIL.** Preferably one that keeps your nursery as stink-free as possible. There are so many types to choose from that *Consumer Reports* actually did a study! First off, are you doing cloth diapers or disposables? Cloth diapers (I salute you!) are fine in a dry pail with a regular garbage bag. The more expensive models for disposables will require their own liners—so you'll be spending as much as $30 a week refilling them. The Diaper Genie is one of the most popular brands, but there are also "touch-free" pails by Graco and Dekor that open when you say "Sesame" (okay, you step on the pedal). A major plus when you have poo all over your hands. Personally, I like the idea of one that boasts odor-eliminating carbon or baking soda. You would not believe what a huge stench such a tiny tush can make. Most diaper pails will run you $25 to $30; it's the refills that get you.

- **A WIPE-WARMER.** Some moms will tell you this is silly—your newborn will do just fine with a moist wipe at room temperature. I beg to differ: My boy hates to feel a cold, wet wipe on his privates in the middle of the night. If he's slightly groggy and needs to be changed, it wakes him up immediately—and he starts screaming like a banshee. The warm wipes comfort and soothe him, and he settles right back down to sleep. I also think the warmer keeps the wipes moist. You can find one for about $20 at Babies "Я" Us. You can use any brand of wipes in it.

- **A FOAM TUB.** I found the Puj Tub to be soft and flexible, and it fits into any sink, so I can give Cree an instant cleanup, and then I can hang the foam tub on the bathroom door until I need it again. What I love most is the fact that it keeps him cradled and secure; I don't have to worry about holding his head up. I have two hands free! At $39.99 on Amazon it's totally worth every penny. For me, it was a lifesaver. My C-section made it hard for me to comfortably bend over a tub and wash the baby; this made it pain-free.

- **A BOUNCY SEAT.** All my mom friends told me to buy a bouncy seat—and now I understand why. With six motions (car ride, kangaroo, ocean, tree swing, ocean wave, and, my fave, rockabye), five speeds, and five built-in nature sounds, my 4moms mamaRoo bouncer is more like a babysitter! Cree is always entertained and soothed in it. I love how it doesn't just jiggle my baby, like less costly bouncy seats that run about $50; it actually mimics natural motion, swaying him from side to side, just like when I rock him in my arms. If you splurge on this, you don't need a baby swing (so you'll save money on that). And more important—you won't need an extra pair of hands! It's about $200 on Amazon.

- **A BOTTLE RACK.** I know how basic this sounds, but I just didn't think about it until my sink and countertops were overflowing with bottles and nipples. There were always some being washed, some drying, some standing around with curdling milk. Enter my bottle rack, a lovely device that allows you to stack, sort, and air-dry it all. Some fold up and have long spikes that hold the bottles in place; others spin like a carousel. For about $10 to $15 at Babies "Я" Us, you too can have one and feel a teeny bit organized while the rest of your life is in chaos.

- **A CONVERTIBLE CRIB.** Since cribs can be supercostly (upward of $5,000 for one that's handcrafted and heirloom quality), you want one that will go the distance and won't need to be replaced as soon as your child is a toddler. Cree's crib actually converts, when he's ready, into a full-size bed. You don't have to spend a fortune on a convertible (also called an all-in-one, a four-in-one, or a lifetime crib); you can find a beautiful one than goes from crib to toddler bed to full-size at Babies "Я" Us for about $300. Remember, you'll also be buying bedding and eventually conversion kits, so budget wisely. I also recommend that you skip the bassinet; you can put the baby in the crib in your room at first, then move him to the nursery once he's sleeping through the night.

- **A PACKABLE PLAYPEN/CRIB.** Mine is from BabyBjörn (Travel Crib Light, $279 on Amazon), and let me tell you, if you are a working mom or are on the road a lot, you cannot live without it. Anytime you need to put your baby down someplace safe and contained, you can set it up in a snap. Cree sleeps in his when he's on the set.

- **A BABY CARRIER.** Carrying your baby strapped to you allows you to eat lunch and take a call! Hands-free parenting! I have a BabyBjörn (about $150 on Amazon), and it's extremely easy to strap on. Some women use a sling-style carrier, where the baby is snuggled in a pouch that goes over one shoulder. I prefer the ones that have a harness over both shoulders and around your waist. The baby is well supported on your chest or on your back. I have a bad back, and I feel like I'm more balanced and comfortable in it.

- **A STROLLER.** By now you must be thinking, Tia, you're missing something. No, it's not my mommy amnesia; it's that strollers are a big deal! They can range from under $100 to several thousand dollars. What are you looking for in a stroller? Size? Something that accommodates all stages? I wanted one that would grow with my baby and be easy for me to push and maneuver. I was lucky enough to receive a Stokke Xplory stroller. This is the smoothest, coolest stroller. It's pricey, I won't lie to you: upward of $1,000. But it is truly the only stroller I will ever need, and it grows with my baby. The alternative is to spend several hundred on a couple of strollers of different sizes and weights. If you do decide to splurge and get a Stokke, you can save some money and skip all the nifty accessories— the parasol, the foot muff, the shopping bag. Not necessary. You don't need to pimp baby's ride unless you want to; he'll be very happy with the basic model.

You may also want to purchase an inexpensive umbrella stroller to toss in the back of taxis or when you're on the run. Look for one you can open and fold with one hand (you are going to be amazed at what you can learn to do with one hand) and sling over your shoulder. Mine is by Chicco and sells for about $69.

Who's Pushing What?

It used to be about the It bag; now it's the It stroller . . . like the one Kourtney Kardashian just had to have (a $750 Orbit). Not all of them are as pricey as the $3,000 Silver Cross pram that Sarah Jessica Parker, Madonna, Victoria Beckham, and Gwyneth Paltrow pushed their precious cargo in. Some stars, such as Jessica Alba, prefer the Maclaren Volo at a frugal $129. While you're stroller shopping, see if you can match the celebrity mom to her brand, and check your answers below.

1. $888 Bugaboo Cameleon	A. Halle Berry
2. $599 Bugaboo Limited Edition Treasu(RED)	B. Salma Hayek
3. $899 Orbit Car Seat System	C. Nicole Kidman
4. $480 Maclaren Double Stroller	D. Kimora Lee Simmons
5. $490 Maclaren Juicy Couture Ryder	E. Gwen Stefani
6. $599 Mountain Buggy	F. Jennifer Garner
7. $399 City Elite Baby Jogger	G. Nicole Richie
8. $319 Chico Cortina KeyFit 30	H. Cate Blanchett
9. $670 Quinny Zapp Buggy	I. Kendra Wilkinson
10. $199 Mutsy Spider Stroller	J. Julianna Margulies

Answers: 1. J; 2. E; 3. F; 4. G; 5. B; 6. C; 7. D; 8. I; 9. H; 10. A

Oh, Baby!

- **MORE THAN A FEW SETS OF NEWBORN CLOTHES AND NEWBORN DIAPERS.** By three weeks, they were already too small. Choose a few onesies that are zero to three months; and spread the word for friends and family to buy you the rest in sizes for three to six months, six to nine months, and even nine to twelve months. Hopefully you won't spend as much time as I did in the exchange line at BabyGap!

- **A BOTTLE WARMER.** You can simply heat some water on the stove and rest the bottle in it, or run it under hot water. I don't recommend microwaving: nuking the bottle can heat it unevenly, so part of the formula or milk can come out scalding hot.

- **A BOTTLE STERILIZER.** A nice idea, but if you have a dishwasher, that'll do just fine. If you're a germaphobe, you can boil the bottles and parts once a week so they're superclean. And if you're afraid of dishwasher residue, just use some soap and water and then give them a good rinse.

You remember what I said about advice, right? If you're reading this having already bought a bottle warmer because you know it'll make your life easier, go for it, Mama! You read what I learned about the wipe warmer for my little man. Your baby may not need or even like a warm wipe. Take what works for you and run with it. Trust your momtuition—it's getting stronger and stronger every day.

What a Girl Wants, What a Girl Needs

My bedroom overfloweth with stretch-mark creams, nursing bras, and breast-feeding pillows—the majority of which were never even used! You are gearing up for a very big day—don't forget to treat yourself to some goodies that will really help you get through the first few weeks and after. Here are my New Mama Must-Haves:

- **A BELLY BAND.** I didn't expect to have rock-hard abs the moment after I delivered—but a belly that shook like jelly? Oh, the horror! My once flat abs were now a jiggly mass of atrophied muscles and fat. A friend highly recommended a belly band. It's like a corset—it sucks it all in. Manufacturers prefer the term *abdominal compression wrap*, and swear that it will restore your body to its beautiful pre-baby shape. I don't know about that—I still look like the Pillsbury Doughboy. But I do think it supports my back and my achy muscles, and made my C-section recovery a little easier. It's also supposed to minimize stretch marks. Tell ya what: I'll settle for the stretch marks as long as my tummy goes back where it belongs!
- **SPANX.** Speaking of sucking it all in . . . I could not live without my Spanx. No matter how many inches I can pinch on my hips, waist, and butt these days, this miracle body shaper shrinks me down to size. While you're pregnant, you can wear the Power Mama ones to support your baby bump. After, I'd spring for the works: high-

waisted, low-waisted, tummy-taming. It's all good. And I swear to you, there ain't an actress on the red carpet who doesn't have them under that skintight dress—even the skinny ones.

- **BREAST-FEEDING PADS.** I was out to dinner with friends the other night in a lovely, flowy boho tunic (sans bra!) and leggings, when I suddenly realized my boob had sprung a leak. I tried stuffing countless tissues and napkins down my shirt, but it was too late: I was like the Fountain of Trevi. Mortified, I excused myself to the ladies' room and vowed I would never go braless and padless again. Most nursing pads are made of a leakproof, ultra-absorbent material. Some even have lanolin on them for sore, cracked nipples (see next item, below). The important thing is they prevent you from embarrassing yourself with ring-around-the-nipple stains. Even if you're not nursing, you can still leak for a few weeks before your milk dries up. You can pick up a box at any baby or maternity store for about $5.

- **NIPPLE CREAM.** After a week of nursing my baby, my nipples looked like they'd been through a war: sore, swollen, red, dry, and cracked. It hurt like hell every time Cree latched on. My nurse at the hospital recommended I try a creamy salve to relieve any itching and pain. There are tons on the market; some are all natural, and some say they're also great for diaper rash (I love multitasking). I recommend you apply whatever nipple balm you choose as soon as the baby is done feeding and leave it on. It took a day or so, but my boobs were much happier.

- **ORGANIC MOTHER'S MILK TEA.** While we're on the subject of breast-feeding—this tea helps your body go with the flow, if you get my drift. Whenever I felt like I was drying up, drinking a cup made my milk come in. The combination of anise, fennel, and caraway supports healthy lactation. It also calms me down and has a little spicy kick to it. Some moms recommend adding a bit of honey if you like your tea sweeter. It costs $7 for a pack of 16 bags on Amazon.com.

- **A ROCKING CHAIR.** At first I thought buying one of these would make me feel like a granny. Not so: I love gently rocking my baby to sleep in the nursery. I find it incredibly peaceful and relaxing for both of us. You can get a soft, cushioned recliner that rocks or an antique wood model (cover the seat with a comfy pillow). I like to wrap us both in a cushy blanket and put on a Baby Mozart CD. Cree and I both veg out.

- **A BREAST PUMP.** I had no idea there were so many choices out there: hand pumps, pumps you can backpack, dual pumps, hospital-grade, piston-driven . . . my head was spinning. The expert at the hospital suggested I consider how often I would be pumping—and where I intended to do it. For example, you'll want a quiet model if you're planning on pumping at work. Double pumps are time savers—they attach to both breasts and work simultaneously. And manual ones are small and discreet—so you can whip it out anywhere, anytime. When it comes down to it, it's a very personal choice. I went with a dual Me-

dela. Ask your friends what models they liked; ask your
OB or a lactation consultant for a recommendation. I
wish they would let you test-drive these things at Babies
"Я" Us before you have to buy (not gonna happen). The
prices range from $35 for a hand model to $1,000 for
hospital-quality. You'll probably wind up spending somewhere in between, around $150 to $300. Look for a model
that comes with bottles you can label with the date and
time pumped. That way you know which milk is fresh
and which bottles are past their prime.

- **NURSING TANK TOPS.** So comfy and convenient. This is basically all I wore for the first weeks after I delivered.
They've got built-in bras and wide, adjustable straps. If
it's cold, you can layer stuff over them. You can work out
in them and even sleep in them. I swear, I never changed
my top and no one was the wiser! I liked the longer,
looser kind, since they covered up my still-swollen stomach. Glamourmom makes a great one in black or white
for $49 (glamourmom.com). The cool thing: It looks like
just a tank, not a nursing top, and the chest stretches with
you as your boobs grow or shrink.

- **A SEXY MATERNITY BRA.** I don't know about you, but an
over-the-shoulder boulder holder is not my idea of
pretty. Just because you're nursing, it doesn't mean you
have to wear ugly undies. There are so many beautiful,
lacy, attractive nursing bras to choose from. And companies like You Lingerie, Cake, and HOTmilk are making
nursing bras (and matching panties!) that are anything

but matronly, in black lace and with little red hearts. I also love the names they give them: Her Tangled Web! Awakened by Her Desire! Now, does that sound frumpy to you?

If It's Free, It's for Me!

The minute you deliver, manufacturers start vying for your business. I was amazed at the loot I left the hospital with: free formula, bottles, nipples and pacifiers, and coupons for tons more. Friends begged me to tell them what I needed and where I was registered. Bring it on!

- **Register for everything.** And I mean everything. Diapers, wipes, ointment, C batteries for the baby monitor. Especially if you know you are having a shower, give your guests loads of options. If they don't want to buy you a dozen burp cloths, at least they'll show up with a gift card. A friend of mine actually registered at three different places: Babies "Я" Us, Target, and Amazon—she also included books and DVDs to stock her baby's nursery shelves. Just make sure everything you ask for is actually for baby or new-mom needs; your friends will be onto you if you register for a new TV.
- **Ask for hand-me-downs.** These gently worn or sometimes unused clothes, shoes, and accessories are a mom's best

friend. Got cousins? College roommates? Neighbors? If they've had kids, they surely want to clean house at some point. Tell them you'll take whatever stuff they care to share that's in good condition. Sometimes people feel awkward offering you their used stuff—so make sure they know you welcome it. You can save a bundle, especially with how quickly babies and toddlers outgrow everything. You can also ask a pal to lend or give you her old maternity clothes—you can prob score some basics and dress them up with new accessories.

- **Send away for samples.** A friend let me in on this one. Parenting magazines, diaper and formula manufacturers, and baby food companies love to send you freebies so that you will become a loyal customer. Often if you sign up at a website, the company will e-mail you coupons, rebates, or gifts on your baby's birthday. Besides the hospital, ask around for samples at your OB, pediatrician's office, or day care center. Last time I was at the doc, I scored several tubes of diaper-rash cream and some great moisturizer for me. Oh, and a few lollipops (although I'm pretty sure I wasn't supposed to take those).

Our First Trip to Babies "Я" Us

Cory and I waited till right before my baby shower to register, and we decided this was a great place to go for everything. Honestly, I think he was more excited than I was.

"Whoa! Check out this baby-crib music player! Tia, you need this? How about that bottle cleaner thingy? Wait... you see this stroller?"

I had been in the store once or twice before to get friends gifts, but now it was my turn. It made it all very real for me. I'll admit, it was overwhelming in the beginning—it took us three and a half hours to make our way through every aisle. There is just so much stuff, and you wonder where it's all gonna go in your house. But they gave me a little pamphlet of essentials, which was a great place to start. We went around, checking off items, throwing in others that were not even listed as must-haves but were just too cute to leave behind. Now I am in this place so often, it's like going to the supermarket!

Ask the OB

My body seems to know that my house is in order. How do I know if these labor pains are false labor (Braxton-Hicks)?

Before labor begins, your body may experience some practice contractions, also known as Braxton-Hicks. They are basically your body's way of getting ready for the Big Day. Real labor contractions usually come at regular intervals, last 45 to 90 seconds, and become more frequent and stronger as time goes by. Braxton-Hicks are usually irregular, not very strong, and may stop with a change of position or activity. If you are sitting, get up and go for a walk, or if you've been walking, lie down and rest. Real contractions will persist and progress; Braxton-Hicks frequently resolve. Another good rule of thumb: If you can have a conversation while you are having a contraction, it's probably not strong enough to be the real deal.

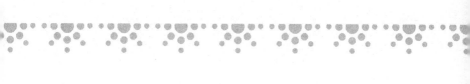

CHAPTER 11

The Big Day

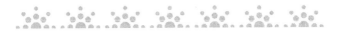

I have run into a little glitch. My amniotic fluid is going down, down, down, and Dr. Kumetz is concerned. So she put me on bed rest. I am not allowed to get up, except to pee. I feel like a prisoner in my own home, and I still have episodes of our _Tia & Tamera_ reality show to shoot. Everyone is working around me. I feel like the five-hundred-pound elephant in the bedroom.

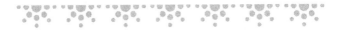

*B*y week thirty-six, the baby was still breech. He was going the wrong way for natural delivery, and he wasn't changing his mind about his direction. I tried everything to turn him. I stood on my head, put clothespins on my toes, even went to a Chinese medicine guy, who put burning herbs on my feet (I kid you not). Nada. Nothing worked. Now what?

"I can try to do an external cephalic version," my OB said. That involved my doctor's physically turning the baby while he was still inside me. I did the research: it didn't sound fun. Most of the comments were things like "OMG! This procedure was the most painful thing I have ever experienced in my life!" and "I wanted a bullet to bite on, it hurt so bad!" On top of all that, the success rate was a mere 50 percent. So I passed; half wasn't enough for me. I told Dr. Kumetz if this was my only choice left, I'd rather go for the C-section, and we agreed to schedule it for June 28, 2011. I tried to look on the bright side.

It was a week earlier than my due date—so I got to see my baby sooner. And I got to get out of bed!

Still, I couldn't help feeling very disappointed. This was not how I imagined myself bringing a baby into this world. I wanted a natural birth, and I wanted to work out right away and get back in shape for my show. A cesarean meant it would be six weeks before I could exercise. I had to come to grips with the fact that I wouldn't look like myself when I started shooting again. I actually had a meeting with one of the producers, Kenny Smith, to explain.

"Tia, we're going to pick up where you left off—the same scene," he told me.

I panicked: "Kenny, I'm not going to be able to get into those same clothes. I'm going to look like a blimp!"

As Hosea had predicted weeks earlier, Kenny assured me they'd work around it—I was kind of hoping he'd offer to hire me a body double, but no go. And it wasn't like they could write my character out for a few weeks while I toned up and slimmed down. It was a major cliff-hanger: a scene where my husband found out I had an abortion.

I went to my appointment with Dr. Kumetz and vented: "Why me? Why couldn't the baby just do a little one-eighty and cooperate?"

"Tia," Dr. Kumetz said, trying to comfort me. "Think of this as your first important life lesson when it comes to parenting. Kids don't always do what you want them to do." I burst into tears. I just lay there for several minutes, sobbing hysterically with my feet in the stirrups. Then I calmed down; it actually felt good to get it off my chest. But I also couldn't help worrying, was this the first of many more frustrating situations to come? Was motherhood going to be a constant struggle? And just how bad was this C-section going to hurt?

I called my friends for support. Paula Patton was my role model: she bounced back from delivery in three months, and went to work shooting *Jumping the Broom*. She looked *amazing* and swore up and down that I would do the same. My other friend Stacy was having a C-section around the same time I was. She talked me off the ledge. "This is my second one, and if I can do it, not once but twice, then you sure can!"

Still, before every OB appointment, I'd say a little prayer that my son would boogie his butt where it belonged and Dr. K would cancel the surgery.

"No matter how he comes into this world, he's yours," my doc reminded me. "Hold on to that thought."

I did. I kept picturing this perfect little baby boy, and counting the days till I could meet him face-to-face. That was also torture. Sometimes I'd notice an expiration date that was beyond June 28 and I'd smile: My baby will be here when I have to toss this OJ. But I was impatient and antsy; I wanted to hold my baby in my arms already.

Finally, the Big Day arrived. I checked into Cedars-Sinai hospital at five-thirty a.m. I was scared as hell. My bag had been packed for weeks: I had my gowns, my extra-strength panty liners, my pump machine, the baby's take-home outfit. I also packed a few hot-mama gowns in beautiful, bright colors and floral prints. And I figured I'd need my full makeup kit—so I tucked that in as well (for the record, I never used it—see p. 202, "Don't Leave Home Without These"). The night before, I didn't sleep at all. I kept looking at Cree's ultrasound pictures and talking to them.

"I can't wait to see you!" I would coo, and Cory would just shake his head. *Get this baby out before my wife winds up in a loony bin . . .*

My mom and my grandma stayed with me that night. I woke up at three a.m.; left the house around five; checked in around five-thirty. I was supposed to get a spacious private birthing suite.

"We're so sorry," a nice hospital employee informed us. "We're renovating, so that's not available."

I shot Cory a look: Do something!

"Well, what *is* available?" my husband asked.

The choices were (a) a $7,000-a-night suite or (b) a tiny room. You can guess where I wound up.

So, as I settled into my bed, my entire family (Mom, Dad, Grandma, and Cory) were cramped in a small corner of my room. I was appalled at how little space there was, but as my mom pointed out, "the love was in the room."

After a few minutes, the nurse came in. Clearly this chick could have used a refresher course in installing an IV line in a patient. She jabbed the back of my hand about a dozen times. When it wouldn't go in the left, she started jabbing the right. I was screaming and crying and blood was spurting everywhere on the bed.

"Okay, fine," she said. "I'll send someone from Anesthesia." She couldn't have done that an hour ago?

Oh, Baby!

She left, and I felt a powerful twinge in my belly.

"Uh-oh," I said to Cory. "I think I'm in labor."

"What?" My husband stared in disbelief. "That's not supposed to happen!"

"Yeah, well, you wanna tell the baby that?"

The contractions started, and they were excruciating and coming closer and closer together. My dad was doing the running sports commentary: "Wow, that was a big one!"

Finally, the anesthesiologist arrived and got the IV in on the first try. They started to prep me and Cory for the surgery. That's when it hit me: It's really happening. They had me put on socks and a scrub cap. I glanced at my husband and made a telepathic plea: "Don't leave me!"

A nurse poked her head in. "It's time! The doctor's here!"

Wait! Stop! I changed my mind! I can't do this! my brain was screaming. *Can we talk this over?*

No such luck; Cory went to get into his scrubs, and I was wheeled on a gurney into the operating room, clutching my iPod. Whoever has been designing the sets for medical dramas over the past ten years is doing a great job—the O.R. looks exactly like it does on TV. Big, sterile, and filled with bright lights and equipment—plus really sharp, pointy tools. One look around, and I was in complete panic mode. *Just breathe, just breathe.*

I could hear the nurse counting all the surgical tools and clanking them onto a tray. "Scalpel one, scalpel two." I hit the Play button on my iPod, and suddenly classical music filled the room over its speaker.

"That's very nice, very relaxing," a nurse told me as soon as my tunes began to play. *Yeah, well I'm happy you're relaxed. I want to get off this table now!*

"We're going to give you an epidural now," she said. Then she held my hand in hers. "Don't worry, it's going to be okay." Thanks, lady, but I don't know you! I want my husband! I want my doctor! I wanna go home!

The anesthesiologist told me to sit up and lean forward into a fetal position. I was squeezing the nurse's hand like a vise, digging my nails into it. I braced myself and . . .

"That's it," he said.

Seriously? That little prick? That was it? It didn't hurt at all. As soon as the medicine went in, I felt a little pressure, and then my legs tingled and felt warm. In two minutes, I couldn't feel anything from the waist down. *Oh, thank you.* They could have sawed my legs off, and I swear I wouldn't have said "ouch" once.

Then I lay back down on the table . . . and they strapped my arms down at the wrists with two buckles. Like a straitjacket! What did they think I was going to do, punch them? Get up and leave? Apparently, it's procedure; they don't want you flailing around and ripping out your IVs.

The nurse started to clean my stomach, swabbing me with Betadine. It felt wet and cold.

"Excuse me, I can still feel this!" I piped up.

Dr. Kumetz was now in the room and I breathed a huge sigh of relief. "Hi, Tia," she said. "You *are* going to feel—just not pain."

If you say so.

Cory came in right after her. I don't know who looked more terrified, him or me. They were draping the blue sheet over me, so I couldn't see any of the action on the other side. "You have the cord-blood-bank kit?" Dr. Kumetz asked.

Oh, no. I'd forgotten it back in my cramped little room. They sent a nurse running down the hall to fetch it while Dr. Kumetz prepped.

 Ask the OB

Is it a good idea to bank the cord blood?

Cord blood is blood that is left in the umbilical cord and placenta after the baby is born. Until recently, this blood was discarded as medical waste. Cord blood contains many stem cells (similar to cells found in bone marrow), which may be frozen for later use in medical therapies such as stem-cell transplants. Cord blood can either be donated for the public or stored privately for the family. If needed, these cells can be thawed and used in either autologous transplant (when someone receives his or her own blood) or allogenic transplant (when a person receives cord blood donated from someone else, such as a sibling, close relative, or anonymous donor).

The most common reason parents consider banking their newborn's cord blood is a family history of diseases that can be treated with bone marrow transplants, such as certain leukemias or lymphomas, and certain inherited anemias. There is lots of research going on to see if these cells may someday be used to treat other disorders, such as spinal cord injuries, cerebral palsy, and stroke. The odds today that the average baby without risk factors will ever use his or her own banked cord blood is considered very low, though no accurate estimates exist at this time. Without a family history of conditions that can be treated today, a good approach is to think of cord-blood banking as a very expensive insurance policy—money you assume you are throwing away because no one will ever need to use it.

"Did anyone do an ultrasound?" I heard her ask. Seemed I wasn't the only one who had forgotten something: None of the docs had checked whether the baby was still breech. Can you imagine if he wasn't?

"This baby better not have turned around—not after I went through all of this!" I moaned.

After confirming yes indeedy, he was still going the wrong way, Dr. K did a pinch test. "Do you feel any pain?" she asked.

"No," I answered. And I truly didn't—just lots of tugging and pressure. I knew that she was cutting me open, and I started to freak out.

"Cory, you have to talk to me," I begged my hubby. "Say something so I am not focused on what's down there."

"Uh, uh, what do you want me to say?" He was watching all these people working and blood everywhere—he was in shock.

Finally, Dr. Kumetz said, "Okay, Tia, you are about to feel some pressure." That was putting it mildly: I felt like I was punched in the stomach! She had to really tug to get the baby out. She told me later she didn't know if the incision was big enough!

I was watching Cory's face upside down the entire time, trying to read him. His mouth was wide open. "Tell me something!" I begged. "Is he okay?"

It was my OB who answered. "He's perfect—and once he was out, he came out running! He has a lot of hair . . . Did you have heartburn?"

The doctors took Cree over to the scale and to the table to clean him up. I heard his cries for the first time and I started bawling—then apologizing to all the surgeons for being so emotional. I have never wailed like that in my life. I couldn't stop. When they swaddled the baby and handed him to Cory, he started crying, too. I have never seen him cry like that, not even on our wedding day. All three of us were blubbering messes—but so, so happy. Then, when Cory put our baby next to me, at least Cree calmed down. My heart opened. I will never, ever forget that feeling: joy, peace, contentment. I just wanted the surgery to be done so I could hold him and rock him and kiss his little cheeks. What they don't tell you is how long it takes to close you up. The actual getting the baby out is lightning-quick, but putting Humpty-Dumpty Mama back together again? A little more complex and time-consuming.

The baby looked up at me. "Yes, I'm the one you've been kicking all this time! I'm your mama!" His eyes were wide open and he was super alert. He was ready to face the world—no napping necessary! I thought he looked like Cory, he was so beautiful. I have never seen anything so beautiful and perfect in my life. And I was so proud of myself for giving birth to him. Hey, look at what Cory and I made! No one else has one like this—he's all mine.

Finally, I was taken into the recovery room so my family could meet him. My parents came in, along with my brothers, Tamera, and my grandma. We were all crying. I was most shocked at the reaction from my younger brother, Tavior. He's a football player at University of California–Davis right now—a huge, muscular guy. When he held Cree for the first time, he just turned to mush and started cooing at him. I loved seeing Tavior's big hands gently cradling something so tiny.

Men are pretty amazing when it comes to babies. From the second he was born, Cory was by the baby's side 24/7. He followed him around the hospital: for his bath, his checkups, his circumcision. He was not going to let Cree out of his sight for a second. It was so sweet; he was already the protective, doting dad. He even put on a second pair of scrubs that said "I'm the Dad!" I marveled at how quickly he fell head over heels in love with our son. There was no fear; no hesitation. He even dove right into changing diapers! Watching my man with our baby made me love and appreciate him even more. I had known he'd be an incredible father one day—and I was right.

I was in the hospital for three days before they turned me loose. I was delighted to get out of there and go home, though parts of me ached and others throbbed. I was so damn constipated—even with stool softeners—that it literally hurt to sit down. I felt like my plumbing was all backed up. Help, Roto-Rooter!

Instead, a very pleasant nurse offered me a hand. Actually a finger.

"I can loosen it up and get it out for you," she said.

"Pardon?"

"I can put on some gloves and take it out—if it's bothering you."

Yes, it's bothering me. But no way is that happening. I thanked her and went home—where I was kind of sorry I had been so hasty.

It was four days before anything came out. And when it did, I felt like I was giving birth. I thought God was playing a joke on me, making me experience all the pain and pushing, since I had skipped that part with a C-section.

I sat in the bathroom for about forty-five minutes, grunting and groaning, huffing and puffing.

Cory was concerned: "You okay in there? Anything I can do?"

Trust me, the last thing you want when you're constipated is an audience.

I finally went—but it was quite an ordeal. My advice: If a kind nurse offers you some assistance . . . don't poo-poo it.

Don't Leave Home Without These

Maybe you'll be like me and have days or even weeks to pack your bag for the hospital. Or maybe you'll have to grab and go. Either way, this checklist will come in handy.

- Insurance and hospital forms
- Birth plan
- 3 pairs of warm socks. I wore mine on the operating table and also while strolling the halls after delivery. Nonskid are the best.
- 2 maternity bras and nursing bras. Even if you're not planning on nursing, the support and leakage protection is helpful.
- Hairbrush and ponytail holders or headbands. Your hair is such a wreck you'll need a way to camouflage.
- Toothbrush and toothpaste
- Deodorant, face wash, moisturizer, makeup. Although I never put any on, you might want to freshen up for visitors. In retrospect, I should have. I'm pretty mortified by how lousy I look in all the pics with Cree those first few days!
- Your MP3 player. I played mine in the O.R. and it soothed my nerves. It's also great when you want to tune out distractions and just concentrate on nursing your little one.
- A journal and a pen. Trust me, you will want to write stuff down. Even if it's just some directions from the nurses on

how to swaddle. I used mine to record my feelings about meeting my beautiful little boy, so I would never forget.

- Camera, film, extra batteries, video recorder. I delegated this to Cory, as I was too busy to be recording the birth!
- Cell phone, charger, and numbers of people to call and share the news. I strongly recommend putting these important peeps on speed dial: your OB, pediatrician, doula, midwife, family, and a few close friends (if they're not already in there). Thanks to the meds, I was in a pleasant haze for a few hours. Dialing more than one letter or number would have been an impossible task.
- 3 or 4 maternity gowns and robes. I made sure I had bright and pretty ones. I didn't care if they got ruined. I did not want to be in a hospital gown with my butt hanging out the back!
- Eyeglasses or contacts (and contact solution). You want to see your baby clearly!
- Money/credit cards. Just in case you need a trip to the vending machine or have to send someone to the cafeteria.
- Breast pump, if you plan to use one. Do not rely on the hospital rentals. Sometimes they're not available and, from what I hear from friends, industrial strength can be pretty painful.
- 6 pairs maternity undies and a box of extra-strength panty liners or sanitary napkins. Trust me, you will need them.
- Massage oils, tennis balls, etc. For your partner to massage you with when you're laboring.

- A little touch of home. A fave pillow, a small picture frame, a lucky charm. Cory brought a pic of his mom, who had passed away, and I wore a red string around my wrist that my grandmother prayed over for protection. Something that's comforting to you and makes your hospital room or birthing suite feel a little less sterile. Do not, I repeat, do not pack your entire bedding set and the contents of your nightstand. Hospital rooms are tiny. And when people send you flowers, balloons, and giant teddy bears, there's barely any room for you and the baby—much less your afghan throw.
- Going-home clothes for both you and the baby. I had an adorable little green two-piece outfit for Cree (with footies!) and some comfy clothes for me. You will not magically shrink to your pre-preggers body after delivery. I was still huge! It takes months for your stomach and uterus to shrink back down where they belong (trust me, my abs look nothing like they once did—and it's been months!). Bring loose, maternity-size clothes and comfy, flat shoes. I wore cute little slippers with bows on them and Hot Mama gowns, which come in bright, cheery colors and patterns. Plus, they allow easy access for nursing (hotmamagowns.com).

Say Cheese!

At the moment, there are probably one thousand pictures of Cree on my iPhone. I am obsessed with taking pics of him. I have snapped every outfit he's ever worn; every gurgle and grin; each time he raised a chubby little fist in the air. Watch out! Mama's got a camera and she knows how to use it! Babies change every day, so make sure you don't miss any of these precious photo ops with your newborn. And I highly recommend you put all these photos into an album, either online or in a scrapbook, so you can share it. One day, your little munchkin will love looking at them, and you don't want them to disappear when you accidentally lose your cell phone or drop it in the toilet (my greatest fear!).

Shots to snap:

1. Bringing baby home from the hospital
2. Baby meeting the family
3. Baby nursing with Mama
4. Baby sleeping
5. Baby's first bath
6. The first time you take baby outside
7. Baby and his or her favorite toy
8. Baby's first smiles
9. Baby's first food (face covered in cereal is always adorable!)
10. Baby's first tooth

Someone to Watch Over Cree

Though many of my friends told me I should hire a baby nurse so I could get a good night's sleep and have time off for good behavior, I didn't want one. I'm selfish. I wanted to spend every moment with my newborn son. I knew that eventually, when I went back to work, I'd have to hire someone to help me care for him. But it was such a huge stress! How could I trust a stranger to take care of my precious baby? How could I let someone I didn't even know into my house, unsupervised, to care for such a tiny infant?

I know a lot of moms feel this way. It's normal. No one knows your baby as well as you do. But that doesn't mean someone can't take care of him. You just have to find the right someone. I was so lucky. My next-door neighbor had her nanny, Ritva, for eleven years, but the kids were getting older. So I hired her and she's amazing. In the beginning, I made sure we were on the same page; she understood how often I wanted Cree changed and fed, and what his usual routine was. I couldn't help feel a pang of jealousy when Ritva picked him up or kissed and cuddled him. I thought, *He's mine! You don't get to do that, I do!* But then I realized how silly that was; I wanted Cree to feel loved and secure all the time, even if I'm not around. And it's unreasonable for me to expect I can be with him 24/7. Sometimes his dad, grandma, aunts, uncles, and babysitter are going to be there, and I had to learn to trust. I'm also very, very lucky that my show, *The Game*, will allow me to bring him to work with me on the set in Atlanta. There, he'll have even more honorary aunts and uncles to dote on him, and I can nurse him between sessions of working.

There will come a time—even if you're a stay-at-home mom—when you have to leave your baby. For most women, it's a huge emotional hurdle to get over. I had to leave Cree for the first time to go do press for *The Game*, and I was a hysterical wreck. I cried and cried, like my heart was breaking in two. I was leaving my best friend, my partner in crime, my homey!

To make me feel a little better, Ritva sent me updates and pictures on my phone throughout the day: how many times he peed and pooped, how many hours he slept, if he burped, you name it. Every time I received a text from her, I was so happy. It made me feel connected to home and him. A friend of mine set up a home video cam so she could log onto a website and see her son playing, eating, or sleeping whenever she felt like it. A simple phone call every hour or two will do the trick, too. Just ask your caregiver to keep you in the loop so you can keep your sanity.

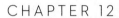

CHAPTER 12

Sleepless Nights and Mommy Milestones

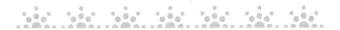

The first time I held my baby in my
arms . . . words can't describe. His eyes
fluttered open and found mine, and we
both stared long and hard. Love at first
sight. He knew instinctively I was his
mama. I couldn't stop looking at him and
marveling, He's mine!

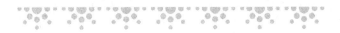

I made a big oopsie on Twitter recently. I wrote, "My son is the love of my life." Poor Cory; I totally forgot him. And I can't even blame it on pregnancy brain anymore. I am just so head over heels with this little boy! Cory forgave me—he feels the same way. Sometimes we just stand over Cree's crib, watching his chest rise and fall as he sleeps. We applaud when he poops and cheer if he douses us in spit-up. It's magic and we're totally under his spell. We actually argue over who gets to feed him when he wakes up every three hours in the middle of the night ("I'll do it—you sleep." "No, I got it!"). Every perfect, tiny finger and toe is a miracle. I can't believe this little person used to be inside me, kicking up a storm. When I'm exhausted and stressed to the breaking point, I just have to pick him up and smell his head (nothing smells more delicious!) and all my anxiety melts away. No one tells you that, either—that someone so tiny could have such power over your heart. They couldn't tell you; you have to feel it for yourself. I love my son so much, it takes my breath away . . .

Experts do a lot of talking about baby milestones: what he should be doing at every new week and month. The day his belly button falls off; the first time he smiles, rolls over, sits up. But I think there were just as many new-mom milestones to mark, some that were joyous, others that were a disaster.

These are the moments I know I will never forget:

The first time I breast-fed. I was in the hospital and the nurses literally threw him on my boob. "Okay, here goes!" I told Cree, hoping he couldn't sense how nervous his mommy was about nursing. I was worried I would be in too much pain because of my C-section, but he latched right on.

"Wow," I said, "that was easy!"

The nurse nodded and pointed to my nipple. "You're lucky," she replied. It was the first time that having torpedo-shaped nipples came in handy. I was so impressed; I thought I had won the lotto! I had heard horror stories of friends who had to hire lactation consultants to get the baby to take. My son was a champ, and I had knockers made for nursing!

My milk production, however, was another thing. It took forever for my milk to come in—nearly three days after I delivered. I was so proud, I demonstrated for the entire family. "You wanna squeeze it?" I asked Tamera. "It's so cool!"

"Eww! Gross!" my twin squealed. "Keep those away from me!"

Ask the OB

When I breast-feed, does everything I eat or
drink wind up in my milk? What should I avoid?

Almost every nursing mother wonders at some point if something she ate caused fussiness, gas, diarrhea, or a rash in her
newborn. Foods that may cause problems for breast-fed babies
include those that contain food additives and dyes, certain gas-
producing foods (such as broccoli, cabbage, and beans), eggs,
nuts, tomatoes, shellfish, chocolate, corn, strawberries, citrus
fruits, onion, garlic, and some spices. Cow's milk in the mother's
diet may cause colicky symptoms in some babies. To decide if a
particular food upsets your baby, eliminate that single food from
your diet for 4 to 7 days and see if the symptoms disappear.
Discuss any dramatic changes to your diet with your doctor or
a nutritionist to be sure you are getting adequate vitamins and
minerals.

Almost every drug or medication makes its way into breast
milk. Some medications appear to have no harmful effects on
your baby, while others are most certainly unsafe. Every new
mother should discuss with her doctor beforehand any medication (prescription or over-the-counter) she plans to take while
nursing.

Caffeine passes into breast milk and may cause your baby to
have an upset stomach and be irritable. Alcohol, including beer,

readily enters breast milk in the same concentration as your blood alcohol level. Since no safe level of alcohol has been established for a breast-fed baby, it is wise to strictly limit your alcohol intake or—even better—not drink at all.

The first time I changed his diaper. My first time was in the hospital, under the watchful eye of a nurse—so I couldn't screw it up. While some people are grossed out, I will tell you I love changing diapers. I get face-to-face with my little one and sing and talk to him while I'm cleaning him up. Disposable diapers make it pretty easy, unless you fail to secure the sticky tabs tight enough. I learned this the hard way. If you don't fasten them well, then baby can spring a leak. One time, shortly after I had gotten Cree home, I was buttoning his onesie when I noticed he was making this face I had never seen before. His nose was wrinkled and his brow was furrowed: he looked like he was concentrating very hard! I picked him up to investigate. Suddenly, the sheets, my clothes, my shoes—everything was covered in poop. I didn't know such a little baby could make such a monstrous poop (he must get that from his dad, not me!). Instead of freaking out, I couldn't help laughing, because we were both such a mess.

Oh, Baby!

The first time I got more than two hours of sleep in a row. The first time Cree slept three solid hours without a whimper, I bolted out of bed and ran to check him in his crib to make sure he was breathing! There he was, sleeping soundly. I was in shock. How did I earn this? At around two months, he was waking me up only once a night. I felt reborn; it's amazing what a little extra sleep, sans interruption, can do for you. I could concentrate, walk straight, and even remember my name. My heart goes out to moms who don't yet have this privilege (my advice: Get the baby on a schedule!). I am so, so grateful that my son is a good sleeper. He must have known how exhausted his mommy was all through the pregnancy and taken pity on me.

The first time I experienced a mommy meltdown. Cree had been home for about two weeks and I was bone-tired. I wasn't getting enough sleep and my room felt like it was caving in on me.

"It's because you stay in here all the time taking care of the baby," Tamera told me, after I complained to her on the phone. "You haven't left the house in fourteen days!"

Well, she was right. Except for the times I took him to the pediatrician, we were home. And for the record, it was more like sixteen days! It felt like I was in the movie *Groundhog Day*: Every morning, I would wake up, feed, change, and burp Cree. He'd doze off; I'd doze off, then the whole cycle would start all over again. I couldn't believe what my life had become. I couldn't remember the last time I'd showered! I felt overwhelmed, and even worse, looming over me was the fact that in six weeks I had to get my act together and get back to work.

I began pacing the floor: What was I going to do? How do other moms do this without becoming walking zombies? How do they make time for the baby and for themselves? I was happy when I got to brush my teeth. I looked in the mirror; OMG, what a mess! I felt frumpy, dumpy, overweight, and overstressed. I wanted to cry; I wanted to scream. But I also didn't want to wake the baby . . .

My first call was to Dr. Kumetz, who assured me these feelings were all normal. What I was experiencing is known as "the baby blues." She told me the transition to motherhood and your new routine can make you anxious and sad, and 80 percent of women experience this during the first few weeks after childbirth.

"You feel overwhelmed and exhausted—and it's all so new to you," my doc told me. "Give yourself some time to adjust. I promise you, they'll go away."

But I needed a little more than medical assurance—so I called the strongest mother I know: my mama.

"How did you do this with twin babies?" I sobbed into the phone. "I can't handle one!"

"Aha . . . now you appreciate what I went through!" She chuckled.

"I'm serious," I pleaded. "I can't do this!"

"You can and you will. You're a lot tougher than you think, Tia."

Maybe it was the drill sergeant talking, but it did get through to me. I vowed to take things one day at a time and not freak out if my baby cried. It didn't mean I was a bad mom; I was just a *new* mom, trying to figure out how to juggle. It took a few weeks, but I got into a groove and I felt so much better!

The first time we went out with the baby. It was like a field trip! I couldn't wait to show him to the world—and frankly, I needed some fresh air myself. So Cory and I made plans with my dad and brother to drive to Hugo's for lunch. We were taking Cree to his first restaurant! I was so excited. Just one small problem: I didn't know it would take an extra two hours to leave the house! I had a ton of baby booty to pack with us: two bottles of breast milk (which I had to pump, taking at least thirty minutes), one bottle of formula (just in case he was still hungry), his car seat/carrier, a blankie, a diaper bag, changing pad, wipes, diaper cream, baby powder, a stack of Pampers, a change of clothes (in case he spit up), and his favorite stuffed giraffe. I stumbled out of the house, barely able to hoist the diaper bag into the trunk of the car.

"You packing for a trip to Europe . . . or lunch?" Cory teased.

"Well, you never know," I insisted. "I just wanna be prepared!"

The first time my baby smiled. Oh, I know people say it's just gas—but I knew better. After just a few days of being home with his mommy and daddy, Cree gave me an adorable, toothless grin. I cried my eyes out. I thought he was looking right into my soul. Did he know who I was? I have a son and I am a mother. I have a huge responsibility for the rest of my life, and I am so, so blessed! After that, all I wanted to do was make him laugh to show him off, so I made silly faces and noises, blew bubbles on his tummy, kissed his toes, anything to get a smiley response. Cory just shook his head: Mama's gone bonkers, baby! And I don't care what those baby books say about babies starting to speak by five or six months—my son is an early learner. I swear, he's trying to talk to me already!

The first time we took a family portrait. Sure, I snapped hundreds of pictures from the moment he was born. But this was a formal portrait—our way of announcing him to the world. It was for *Us Weekly*, when he was just two months old, and it felt so amazing! Cree sat in my lap and posed like a pro. He made me so proud. Cory was there, too, and it felt amazing: This is our family. The three of us. We're a unit now. I can't wait to send out Christmas cards: Meet the Hardricts!

The first time my hubby and I went on a date night . . . post-baby. I was dying to spend some quality time with Cory, just us two. My mom was amazing—she came over every single weekend to help with the baby, and after a few weeks, we finally decided it was time to enjoy a little grown-up playdate. I was nervous about leaving Cree, although I knew he was in the best of hands. But every mama muscle in my body was crying out for him. And if that wasn't bad enough, my boobs ached and reminded me it would soon be time to nurse.

I got cleaned up, put on a pretty dress, and we went to dinner and a movie—nothing fancy. It felt so nice to hold Cory's hand, gaze into each other's eyes, and talk. And you know what we talked about. The baby! Seriously, we spent most of our meal showing each other photos on our phones of him. It made us both laugh. We are such proud parents, we can't help ourselves.

I did have to remind myself that every date night can't be about Cree. The point of getting out with your partner is to show him some attention.

A lot of men feel neglected when the baby comes along; it's a little like being the third wheel. Suddenly, all your attention and affection, which had been only for your man, is focused on this tiny little being. So you have to make an extra effort to include your guy. Involve him in the whole process, every step of the way. There is no baby task Cory won't tackle, from spit-up, to poopy diapers, to two a.m. feedings. We are quite a team, and my mom is so impressed that I found myself a husband who wants to be a daddy 110 percent. I know that later on in life, no matter what happens, we'll be able to handle the tough stuff together. From toddler to teen years (God help us!). And I made Cory a promise that, as much as I love our son, I will always remember he was there first!

Ask the OB

I heard you have to be careful after you've delivered—you're extra fertile and can get pregnant again really easily. True?

You're not necessarily extra fertile right after delivery, but it is possible to get pregnant right away. Many couples are distracted by caring for a newborn, and had not been worried about contraception for at least the previous 9 months, so it's not the first thing on their minds. Ready or not, however, ovulation can potentially occur as soon as 6 weeks after delivery! Breast-feeding decreases fertility but does not eliminate it completely. It's also important to know that you will ovulate before your first period, so just because you are not bleeding monthly, that doesn't mean you can't get pregnant. It is therefore important to come up with a good contraceptive plan, even before delivery, so you are not "caught with your pants down."

Help, I Want My Body Back!

I was in shock when, a month after delivering, I looked down at the saggy tire that was still around my middle. I see all these celebs with flat abs days after giving birth. Well, it didn't happen to me! I was in an elevator, and a lady asked, "Ooh, when are you due?" I grimaced: "No, actually, I had the baby." Ugh.

Oh, Baby!

Women feel the pressure to lose the baby weight right away—and it's even worse if you're someone like me who is in the public eye. It's like my fans and the media expected me to pop out a kid and pose in a bikini a week later. You gotta be kidding.

"You know they're gonna want you back on the show in lingerie ASAP," my cast mate Wendy reminded me.

"I know, I know," I moaned. "This is so unfair!"

First of all, I spent the last part of my pregnancy with my butt glued to the bed. Translation: No exercise. Then I had a C-section and a miserable, painful recovery for six weeks. No exercise again. My trainer, Jeanette, assured me that I could and would get back in shape. She motivated me during my pregnancy to stay active, and I'm proud to say that, with her help, two months after I delivered, I had lost thirty-seven of my fifty-seven pregnancy pounds!

I know a lot of stars train like Serena Williams and starve themselves back to a size zero in no time. Not me. I like to eat too much. My thing is this: The time you spend working out and trying to lose the weight instantly is the time you could be bonding with your baby. The more time you spend in the gym is more time you're spending away from your baby. So take your time. Don't rush, and listen to your instincts. Take it one day at a time. Everything is always changing. And please don't compare yourself to Victoria Beckham, Miranda Kerr, or even me. A healthy weight loss is four to five pounds a month. Thanks to food poisoning, a yeast allergy, and very long days on the set, I dropped from 177 pounds to 136 pounds in about three months. I recommend my diet and exercise routine but not the other complications! Just remember, this isn't a race to get into your skinny jeans again. It's a plan to stay healthy for your baby, who needs you. If you starve yourself, you're not going to be able to nurse or care for your child.

I remember when I first started nursing at home, I was feeling very faint and weak. My nutritionist, Melissa, said, "Tia, every single time you pump or breast-feed, you have to have protein. Keep almonds next to you and boil some eggs and put them in the fridge."

It wasn't as though I was trying to starve myself; I was just too busy and tired to eat.

"You don't want to wind up back in the hospital, dehydrated or malnourished," she insisted. "Cree needs his mama!"

Thanks to Melissa, I am now focused on eating healthy and cutting down on carbs (bye-bye, sourdough bread!), so I have more strength and energy. Plus, I made it my business to squeeze in a workout whenever I could, even if it was just climbing up stairs instead of taking an elevator, or strapping Cree in a baby carrier and walking around the neighborhood. As time went on, the scale started to go down and I began to feel like my old self. So many of my fans were e-mailing me: "How did you do it?" It helped that I was swollen like a balloon and looked huge on *Tia & Tamera*. My "After" pics are svelte in comparison. But I assure you, it wasn't like it just melted off. It took a lot of discipline, and support from my friends. The other day, I was out to dinner with Hosea for his birthday, and he actually slapped my hand as I reached into his plate for some of his dinner.

Oh, Baby!

"Hey . . . drop it! You're not pregnant anymore!" he warned me.

I grumped, but he was right. And I have definitely had to curb my love of cupcakes. It's hard to reprogram your brain to think you're eating for one again! But I figure the one thing I can control is what I put in my mouth.

And don't believe moms who tell you that if you breast-feed, you'll lose all your baby weight. I did not find that one to be true. The average mom will make about twenty-four to twenty-eight ounces of breast milk a day. It takes about five hundred calories to make that much milk. Some of those calories come from fat stored during the pregnancy or previously, and some come from the mother's daily nutrition. So you have to eat right as well as move to really shed the weight.

Since I have the attention span of a flea and basically hate to work out on machines, I discovered Zumba. I love my class, and I really don't think of it as exercise—it's so much fun. It's a form of Brazilian dance, so it's very sexy! It helps me feel like the hot mama I am! I'm constantly shaking my booty and my hips, shimmying my shoulders. The music is red-hot Latin and it gets my blood bumping. You can find a class in your area, or order a DVD and boogie off the belly flab at home. If I can't get to a class in Atlanta when filming *The Game*, I do my moves at home while Cree is napping. You can also check out "Love Zumba" on YouTube for videos that teach the moves by breaking them down at a slow tempo. Just remember that some Zumba workouts can be pretty intense; make sure you talk to your doctor before starting any home fitness routine.

Do the Best You Can

No parent is perfect. I have to remind myself of this each and every day, because I want to do everything right for my baby and I beat myself up if I don't. There's a huge learning curve when you're a first-time mom. I wish that I could figure things out faster (how do you fold this stroller?) and understand the language of babies better. Tamera and I were out for a walk a few weeks ago and every time we'd stop to catch our breath, Cree would start to wail.

"What's wrong, little man?" I asked. As if he was gonna tell me at two months old. So we did a little experiment. I started walking again and he stopped crying. Then I stopped dead in my tracks and the bawling began. Took some more steps . . . no more tears.

"He wants us to keep moving. He's checkin' out the scenery!" I told my sis.

"How did you know that?" Tamera marveled.

I didn't. I just used my momtuition and was patient with both my baby and myself.

That's the big lesson here: You're human. You can't be expected to know everything off the bat. You're gonna screw up (need I remind you of the poopy diaper explosion?). You're going to feel guilty, anxious, and overwhelmed. It comes with the territory.

En route to Atlanta, I phoned our pediatrician, freaking out.

"I think I see a blister on the back of the baby's throat!" I told her. "Oh my God! What is it? Is he sick?" This was all I needed. I was stressed out enough about having to move all our things—and Cree's things—to Atlanta for months to shoot my show. And to top things off, Cory wasn't coming with me! He got a great role in a movie with John Malkovich that was filming in Quebec. He felt awful that we'd be apart and that he couldn't kiss his son good night, and I felt equally awful that though a nanny would help me during the day, I'd be without the partner I'd grown used to tag-teaming with on midnight feedings.

The pediatrician could hear the fear and desperation in my voice.

"Well, is he crying? Does he feel warm?" the doc asked. "Does he seem tired or cranky?"

I looked at Cree, who was beaming from ear to ear. "No, he seems fine."

"Then he probably *is* fine," she told me. "If he wasn't, he'd let you know it." Turns out it was some formula stuck back there. Who knew?

Confession time. If I was a neurotic and a control freak pre-pregnancy, I am ten times as bad now. But I've learned to prioritize. I used to be about checking all the items off my to-do list. Now I rank them by necessity and force myself to live with those decisions, even if they're not neat and tidy and ideal. For example: What can I do with a free hour? Wash the dishes, run on the treadmill, or go to the pharmacy and pick up more formula. I weigh my options and (of course!) the baby wins out. Formula it is! I prioritize and find time later that day to squeeze in a quick fifteen minutes on the treadmill while watching the evening news. As for the dishes, well, they're just gonna have to sit in the sink for a few more hours. No biggie. I don't have to be Superwoman. I can set my limits and say no. I recently had to explain to my publicist, Jordyn, that I don't move as fast as I used to.

"I meant to e-mail you back, but then Cree started crying and I had to feed him," I explained. I also can't do every interview or appearance Jordyn or my show would like me to do, especially not at night. From nine to five I will work like a dog. But after that, it's family time. No cell phones, no e-mails, no distractions. Those are my rules. Things may not always be this way, but this is how it has to be while I figure out how to juggle being both a mom and a working actress. Thank God I have such great people around me who understand. I know not everyone is this lucky.

What I Learned from My Mom About Being a Mom

The one person who can understand this whole working-mom thing better than anyone is my mom. Because she and my dad were stationed overseas, she gave birth to me and Tamera in Germany, away from her whole family back home in Miami. None of the doctors knew English and they didn't have her health records on file. My dad actually fainted during the delivery (big help!), and the only thing he remembers was the doctor saying *"Scheisse!"* because he was surprised to discover my mom was having twins.

My mother, Marlene, has been the person I've talked and

cried to about going back to work. When Tamera and I were babies, my mom had to put us in day care, and it broke her heart; she knows what I'm feeling these days.

She made a lot of sacrifices for her kids. As we got older, she quit her job for us so we could be in show business, and dedicated fifteen years of her life to our careers. She took us to dance and acting classes and auditions and commercials and pageants . . . it was endless. Now I see how strong she was. She came from nothing. She lived with ten brothers and sisters in a tiny apartment. She's a survivor, a fighter, and I am in awe of how she handled it all. I was raised with discipline, but I know that discipline is a form of love. She would tell us when we came home from school, "Do your homework and your chores . . . then you can go out and play." She believed in us, and she now tells me, "Pay attention to your child as he grows up. See what he's good at and what he gravitates toward, and nurture that passion."

I couldn't ask for a better role model in the mama department; mine is amazing in every way, and I have some pretty massive footsteps to follow in. She's generous, kind, compassionate, strong, courageous, and loving beyond the bounds of this world. If I can be half as good a mama, and do it with such style and grace . . . Cree will be one lucky little boy.

Slowly and surely, I'm getting my groove back, and you will, too. It takes time. It takes patience. It takes strength, because people are going to assume you can just pick up where you left off. I used to think, "I want to have it all." Now I just think, "I want to be together." Or maybe, "I want to be sane!"

As Cree gets bigger (thirteen pounds at two months . . . he's huge!) and older, it'll become a lot easier, because he won't need the constant attention. One day there won't be bottles to fill or diapers to change. If I told you I was looking forward to that, I'd be lying. I love this mommy-and-me time; I love loving my baby and holding him in my arms. I love that my little munchkin monopolizes my life! The time goes by so fast; don't rush it. Savor every second. This was something a lot of my friends told me when I got pregnant, and I can tell you, without any doubt, it's absolutely true. They're babies for only the blink of an eye. This is what you've worked so hard for. You've carried your child for nine months; you've delivered him or her into this big world. Don't sweat the small stuff. Count your blessings each and every day—you're this baby's one and only mama. And I'll tell you something else: I want to have more. I can't wait to get pregnant again and have another baby! Remember when Cory was begging for baby number one? Now he thinks I need my head examined.

"Tia, after all you put me through, can you at least give me a little time?"

But I just can't help it: How often do you get to be part of a miracle? And now that I've been through it, I know a little bit more of what to expect, and I know how wonderful the end result is. I've become quite the pregnancy and baby expert among my newly preggers pals, and there are a lot of them. My stylist, Alexis, and two of the ladies in The Game's wardrobe department are expecting. I think I either inspired them, or there's something in the water (probably both!). And you should see the e-mails and Facebook queries I am getting: everyone wants my new-mama insight. I am so excited to give it, and to talk to any mom I meet. Seriously, I stop women with strollers in Starbucks and start conversations. I'm so glad to be a part of this sisterhood and I'm incredibly curious!

Beyond the technical stuff—such as how many times your baby will poop a day (for the record, as many as eight to ten times!)—women are always asking me if motherhood will change them. Well, I am certainly not the same person I was pre-Cree. I'm seeing through my son's eyes, and everything is so exciting, big, and beautiful. Tamera teases me that I've gone all warm and fuzzy and sentimental (and who's the one who put her dog in the wedding party?). Last year, when I was working in Atlanta on *The Game*, I never once left my hotel room. I swear, all I did was go to work and come home to sleep. But now that I have Cree, I'm going everywhere, taking him to the botanical gardens, the aquarium, out to restaurants. He's my date! I never used to get excited at the prospect of seeing a giant whale hanging from the ceiling, but now I can't wait to show it to my baby boy. I want to see his little eyes get round as saucers as he contemplates, "What *is* that?"

Am I a changed person? Totally. Changed for good. And trust me, all the headaches and heartburn you suffered . . . you kind of forget about it (unless, like me, you write it all down!). No one can tell you what this feels like. You can't put it into words. You can't know until you're a mom. But I can tell you this: Having a child is the greatest thing I have ever done in my life.

Oh, baby, it's been quite an adventure, and so worth it.

AFTERWORD

*S*ince this book was first published in May 2012, so much has happened in my life! First of all, my sweet pea Cree is officially fifteen months old. I cannot get over how fast babies grow and change. Every day he does something new and wonderful to amaze me. There have been so many moments, it's almost impossible for me to list them all. But here are a few of my faves:

- The first time Cree laughed. He was just six months old. It wasn't just a little giggle, but a full belly laugh! Blowing bubbles just cracks him up. Even when he's in the tub, I'll put the bubbles in my hand and blow and he laughs himself silly.
- His first word at seven months. Yeah, it was "Dada." I'm like, "I've been with you every single day, changing your diaper and breast-feeding you, and you pick HIM?" But it didn't matter—it was amazing to hear my baby communicate.
- When he knew what a cow and a dog say. He just LOVES books—I will read him not one, but about seven before bed. He follows the pages as I turn them, and he knows how to point to a cow and go "moo." He is just so smart (and I am not biased)!
- His first steps. He started walking exactly two days after his birthday. I cried and I cried and I cried. You start to

realize your baby is growing up, and you're like, "Slow down! Be little for just a little longer!"

- The first time he gave me a hug. He just reached out his arms and threw them around my neck. He was about eleven months old. I love that he can express love. He gives hugs and kisses to his friends, family, and his teddy bear. It is the sweetest thing!

- His first tooth. He was seven months old. Now he has eight teeth, so he is eating anything and everything. They ask in restaurants, "Do you need to see the kid's menu?" I say, "Nah, bring him the full-size portion!" He loves salmon, seaweed, miso soup, and tofu. But his favorite thing in the world is meatballs. He tried them first when we were in New York City promoting the book, and they make him go wild when he sees them on the plate! My little man can eat! He's huge: he's 95th percentile across the board—height, weight, head, all over. Maybe he'll be a football player like my brothers?

I'm still keeping my journal, taking lots of notes so I'm prepared for baby number two and whatever motherhood may throw my way. My motto is, "Take it all one day at a time." I kind of let Cree lead me and I go with the flow. I'm still learning every single day. I'm a first-time mom, so I think I'll be a little more relaxed with the second baby (no bun in the oven yet . . . but we're talking about trying soon). I am an attachment parent and I'm proud of it! But Corey has me beat—he is a helicopter dad, no doubt about it. When Cree falls, Corey rushes to pick him up. I tell him, "Let him try to get up on his own!" but Daddy doesn't want to see his little boy get a boo-boo!

My sissy Tamara is now also expecting, so that has been an incredible experience for both of us. She read this book and told me her favorite chapter was "Hot Mama," the style one. She also owes me a big thank-you for helping her deal with those third-trimester queasies. I think pregnancy nausea must be hereditary, because she was just as miserable as I was. I taught her my tricks (ginger candy and ginger tea). I also know she took my advice about what you need and don't need in your nursery. Hers looks EXACTLY like mine!

I'm excited to imagine what the next few years will hold for me professionally and personally. I can't wait for Cree to grow and learn, but I also hope he never gets too old for his Mama's snuggles and kisses! I am savoring every minute. I am working on so many new future projects, including a musical (yes, I sing and dance!) called *Mistletones* for ABC Family and a pilot where I get to play a mom for the first time.

I want to thank everyone who reached out to me this first year of mommyhood. I love your advice. I love your questions. I love hearing your stories!

ACKNOWLEDGMENTS

I'd like to thank . . .

My husband, who has been my rock and the shoulder I needed to cry on through those sleepless nights.

Cree Taylor Hardrict, my joy, life, and reason. My baby boy allowed me to understand the true meaning of unconditional love. He is my motivation, every day, to be a better person.

My mom and dad: without them and God, I wouldn't even exist—wink, wink.

My brothers, who continue to show me on a daily basis what I get to look forward to with having a son (they both equally hate my wet kisses).

My twin sister, Tamera Mowry, with whom I shared the womb and who never once said I looked fat, when I did in fact gain sixty pounds.

My best friend, Jessica Laskey, who laughed along with me and not at me.

My book collaborator, Sheryl Berk, for making this such a great, fun experience.

My assistant, Alexis Felder.

The cast, crew, and creative team of *The Game*. Thanks for being so supportive and for having my back.

Katherine Latshaw at The Literary Group, and the great team at Avery, especially my editor, Cara Bedick, editorial director Megan Newman, and publisher Bill Shinker.